# OWEN HUNTER

# The Age-Defying Nutrition Plan

First edition

This book was professionally typeset on Reedsy.
Find out more at reedsy.com

# Contents

# INTRODUCTION

Aging is an inevitable part of the human experience, yet the journey through the golden years need not be one of decline and diminishing vitality. In today's world, where life expectancy continues to rise and the desire for longevity is at an all-time high, we have a unique opportunity to redefine the aging process and embrace a future of vibrant, youthful health. The key to unlocking this potential lies in the power of nutrition.

As we grow older, our bodies undergo a complex series of physiological changes that can have far-reaching consequences on our overall well-being. Organs and tissues gradually lose their efficiency, cellular function becomes impaired, and the risk of age-related diseases, such as heart disease, cancer, and Alzheimer's, increases significantly. This natural progression of aging is often accompanied by a decline in physical strength, cognitive abilities, and overall quality of life – a fate that many have resigned themselves to accept.

However, the narrative of aging does not have to be one of inevitability. Groundbreaking research in the fields of nutrition, genetics, and regenerative medicine has revealed that we have a far greater degree of control over our aging trajectory than previously thought. By making strategic dietary choices and incorporating specific nutrient-dense foods into our daily lives, we can actively combat the underlying mechanisms of aging and maintain a level of vitality that defies the conventional wisdom of growing old.

The Age-Defying Nutrition Plan is a comprehensive guide that will empower you to take charge of your aging process and unlock the boundless potential of a youthful, vibrant life. Through a deep dive into the latest scientific evidence and time-tested nutritional practices, this book will equip you with the knowledge and tools necessary to slow down the aging clock, optimize your body's natural defenses, and cultivate a profound sense of well-being that transcends the limitations of chronological time.

At the heart of this transformative approach lies the recognition that nutrition is not merely a means to sustain our physical bodies, but a powerful lever for influencing the very fundamental processes of aging itself. By strategically nourishing our cells with a synergistic blend of macro- and micronutrients, we can support the body's innate regenerative capacities, combat oxidative stress, and foster a state of dynamic equilibrium that enables us to thrive well into our golden years.

Throughout the pages of this book, you will discover the scientific rationale behind an age-defying nutrition plan, explore a vast array of nutrient-dense superfoods and their rejuvenating properties, and learn practical strategies for integrating these powerful dietary principles into your daily life. From the gut-brain axis and the role of the microbiome in longevity, to the transformative power of fasting and the synergistic effects of exercise, you will embark on a journey of self-discovery that will forever change the way you approach the aging process.

Imagine a future where you move through the world with a spring in your step, a clarity of mind, and a vibrant glow that defies your chronological age. This is not merely a fanciful dream, but a very real possibility within your grasp. By embracing the strategies and insights presented in The Age-Defying Nutrition Plan, you will unlock the keys to longevity and reclaim your birthright to a life of youthful vitality.

As we delve into the fascinating world of age-defying nutrition, it's important to acknowledge that aging is a universal experience shared by all of humanity. However, the manner in which we approach this journey can vary greatly. For some, the prospect of growing older may evoke feelings of anxiety, dread, or a sense of powerlessness in the face of an inevitable decline. Others may view aging as a natural progression, accepting its challenges with grace and equanimity.

Regardless of your current mindset, this book aims to shift the paradigm and empower you to reframe your relationship with the aging process. By nurturing an "ageless mindset" – a steadfast belief in your ability to shape your own destiny and defy the limitations of time – you will cultivate a profound sense of agency and self-determination that will serve as the foundation for your journey towards vibrant, youthful health.

Throughout this transformative exploration, we will challenge the conventional wisdom that aging is a one-way street of decay and deterioration. Instead, we will embrace a vision of aging as a dynamic, multifaceted process that can be actively influenced and even slowed down through the intentional application of strategic nutritional practices.

Get ready to embark on an exhilarating adventure that will redefine your understanding of aging and equip you with the knowledge and tools necessary to achieve a level of vitality that defies the passing of the years. The Age-Defying Nutrition Plan is your roadmap to a future of boundless energy, sharp cognitive abilities, and a radiant, youthful glow that will inspire and captivate all who encounter you.

The time has come to reject the notion that growing old means growing weak, and to embrace a bold new vision of aging that celebrates vibrant health, unwavering mental clarity, and a zest for life that knows no bounds. Join me on this transformative journey, and together, we will unlock the secrets to age-defying nutrition and reclaim your birthright to a life of youthful vitality.

# CHAPTER 1

Chapter 1: The Fundamentals of Longevity Nutrition

As we embark on our journey towards vibrant, youthful health, it's essential to establish a solid foundation of understanding around the core principles of longevity nutrition. In this chapter, we will delve into the fundamental macronutrients and micronutrients that play a pivotal role in combating the aging process and supporting overall well-being.

Macronutrients: The Building Blocks of Life

At the most basic level, the food we consume can be broken down into three primary macronutrients: carbohydrates, proteins, and fats. While each of these macronutrients serves a unique and vital function within the body, it is the delicate balance and synergistic interplay between them that holds the key to unlocking the secrets of longevity nutrition.

Carbohydrates: Fuel for Cellular Rejuvenation

Carbohydrates are the body's primary source of energy, providing the fuel necessary to power the countless metabolic processes that sustain life. However, not all carbohydrates are created equal when it comes to supporting healthy aging.

The carbohydrates found in processed, refined foods – such as white bread, pastries, and sugary snacks – can contribute to a host of age-related problems, including insulin resistance, chronic inflammation, and oxidative stress.

These "empty calories" offer little to no nutritional value and can ultimately lead to weight gain, metabolic dysfunction, and an increased risk of age-related diseases.

In contrast, complex carbohydrates found in whole, unprocessed foods – such as vegetables, fruits, whole grains, and legumes – are a rich source of essential vitamins, minerals, and fiber. These nutrient-dense carbohydrates not only provide sustained energy but also support the body's natural detoxification processes, regulate blood sugar levels, and promote the growth and repair of healthy cells.

By favoring complex carbohydrates over their refined counterparts, you can harness the power of these nutrient-rich foods to support cellular rejuvenation, combat oxidative stress, and maintain metabolic balance – all of which are crucial components of an age-defying nutrition plan.

Proteins: The Building Blocks of Tissue Repair and Regeneration

Proteins are the fundamental building blocks of the human body, responsible for the construction, maintenance, and repair of tissues, organs, and cells. As we age, our bodies' ability to efficiently synthesize and utilize proteins can diminish, leading to a gradual decline in muscle mass, strength, and overall functionality.

To combat this age-related protein deficit, it is essential to prioritize high-quality, bioavailable protein sources in your diet. Animal-based proteins, such as lean meats, poultry, fish, and eggs, are excellent sources of complete proteins, containing all the essential amino acids necessary for optimal tissue repair and regeneration.

For those following a plant-based or vegetarian/vegan diet, it is important to carefully combine different protein-rich foods, such as legumes, nuts, seeds, and whole grains, to ensure the complete amino acid profile is obtained. This strategic approach to plant-based protein consumption can help maintain muscle mass, support immune function, and promote cellular rejuvenation – all of which are crucial for healthy aging.

Additionally, the timing and distribution of protein intake throughout the day can also play a significant role in supporting longevity. Consuming smaller, evenly spaced protein-rich meals or snacks can help optimize muscle protein synthesis and prevent the age-related loss of lean muscle mass.

Fats: The Forgotten Ally in Longevity Nutrition

For decades, fat has been unfairly demonized as the primary culprit behind a host of age-related health issues, including heart disease, obesity, and cognitive decline. However, the latest research has revealed a far more nuanced and complex role for dietary fats in the context of longevity.

Healthy, unsaturated fats – such as those found in avocados, nuts, seeds, and fatty fish – are now recognized as essential components of an age-defying nutrition plan. These beneficial fats serve a multitude of functions, from supporting brain health and cognitive function to regulating inflammation and promoting cellular repair.

Monounsaturated fats, such as those found in olive oil and avocados, have been shown to improve insulin sensitivity, lower cholesterol levels, and reduce the risk of cardiovascular disease – all of which are critical factors in maintaining youthful vitality as we age.

Polyunsaturated fats, particularly the omega-3 fatty acids found in fatty fish and walnuts, play a pivotal role in supporting brain function, reducing inflammation, and even helping to stave off age-related cognitive decline, including Alzheimer's disease.

In contrast, the consumption of unhealthy, saturated and trans fats – often found in processed foods, fried items, and baked goods – can contribute to a host of age-related problems, including heart disease, obesity, and metabolic dysfunction. By minimizing the intake of these harmful fats and prioritizing the consumption of nutrient-dense, unsaturated fats, you can unlock a powerful ally in your quest for longevity.

Micronutrients: The Longevity Catalysts

While macronutrients provide the fundamental building blocks for cellular function and tissue repair, it is the intricate interplay of micronutrients – vitamins, minerals, and antioxidants – that truly catalyze the age-defying process. These essential nutrients, often found in abundance within whole, unprocessed foods, play a crucial role in supporting the body's innate regenerative capacities and combating the underlying drivers of aging.

Vitamins: The Guardians of Cellular Health

Vitamins are essential organic compounds that the body requires in small quantities to perform a wide range of vital functions. From supporting immune function and regulating hormone levels to promoting skin health and maintaining cognitive abilities, these powerful micronutrients are indispensable in the fight against the ravages of time.

Vitamin C, for instance, is a potent antioxidant that helps neutralize free radicals, reduce inflammation, and support the production of collagen – a crucial component of healthy skin, joints, and blood vessels. Vitamin E, on the other hand, is a fat-soluble antioxidant that protects cell membranes from oxidative damage, enhancing the body's ability to repair and regenerate.

Vitamin D, often referred to as the "sunshine vitamin," plays a pivotal role in supporting bone health, immune function, and even mood regulation – all of which are essential for maintaining a vibrant, youthful life. Vitamin B complex, comprising a suite of essential B vitamins, is instrumental in converting food into energy, supporting nervous system function, and promoting healthy red blood cell production.

By ensuring that your diet is rich in a diverse array of vitamin-rich foods, you can harness the power of these longevity-boosting micronutrients to support cellular health, combat oxidative stress, and foster a state of dynamic equilibrium within the body.

Minerals: The Orchestrators of Physiological Harmony

Minerals are inorganic compounds that the body requires in small quantities to perform a wide range of essential functions, from regulating fluid balance and nerve transmission to supporting bone density and enzymatic activity.

Calcium, for instance, is a crucial mineral for maintaining strong, healthy bones, which is particularly important as we age and face an increased risk of osteoporosis and fractures. Magnesium, on the other hand, is a versatile mineral that plays a key role in energy production, muscle function, and the regulation of blood pressure – all of which are vital for preserving youthful vitality.

Zinc is another essential mineral that supports immune function, wound healing, and the production of DNA – all of which are critical for combating the age-related decline in cellular regenerative capacity. Selenium, a trace mineral with powerful antioxidant properties, has been shown to help protect the body against oxidative stress and support thyroid function, which can deteriorate with age.

By incorporating a diverse array of mineral-rich foods, such as leafy greens, nuts, seeds, and lean proteins, into your diet, you can ensure that your body has the necessary building blocks to maintain physiological harmony and promote longevity.

Antioxidants: The Defenders Against Aging

Antioxidants are a special class of micronutrients that play a pivotal role in the fight against the ravages of aging. These powerful compounds work by neutralizing harmful free radicals and reactive oxygen species, which can otherwise wreak havoc on cellular structures, leading to oxidative stress, inflammation, and an increased risk of age-related diseases.

Carotenoids, such as beta-carotene and lycopene, are potent antioxidants found in vibrant, pigmented fruits and vegetables. These compounds have been shown to support eye health, enhance immune function, and even reduce the risk of certain cancers.

Polyphenols, another class of antioxidants abundant in berries, green tea, and red wine, have been lauded for their ability to combat inflammation, improve cognitive function, and support cardiovascular health.

Coenzyme Q10, a vital antioxidant produced naturally by the body, plays a crucial role in energy production and has been linked to improved heart health and enhanced athletic performance – both of which are essential for maintaining a youthful, vibrant lifestyle.

By prioritizing the consumption of a diverse array of antioxidant-rich foods, you can equip your body with a powerful defense against the ravages of time, helping to preserve cellular integrity, reduce inflammation, and support overall longevity.

The Synergistic Power of Macronutrients and Micronutrients
    While the individual roles of macronutrients and micronutrients are essential in the pursuit of longevity, it is the synergistic interplay between them that truly unlocks the transformative potential of an age-defying nutrition plan.

By thoughtfully combining nutrient-dense whole foods that provide a balanced blend of carbohydrates, proteins, fats, vitamins, minerals, and antioxidants, you can create a symphony of nourishment that supports the body's natural regenerative processes, reduces inflammation, and promotes overall well-being.

For instance, pairing a lean protein source, such as grilled salmon, with a side of roasted sweet potatoes and a green salad adorned with avocado and a drizzle of olive oil, creates a nutritional powerhouse that not only satisfies the palate but also nourishes the body on a cellular level. The omega-3 fatty acids in the salmon work synergistically with the antioxidants in the greens and the complex carbohydrates in the sweet potatoes to combat oxidative stress, support brain function, and regulate blood sugar levels – all of which are critical for slowing the aging process.

By embracing this holistic, nutrient-dense approach to eating, you can harness the collective wisdom of macronutrients and micronutrients to unlock the secrets of longevity and embark on a journey of vibrant, youthful health.

In the chapters that follow, we will delve deeper into the specific nutrient-rich foods, dietary strategies, and lifestyle practices that can help you put these fundamental principles of longevity nutrition into action, empowering you to defy the limitations of time and reclaim your birthright to a life of boundless vitality.

# CHAPTER 2

Chapter 2: Anti-Aging Superfoods: Fueling Your Body's Defenses

In the quest for vibrant, youthful health, the foods we choose to nourish our bodies with play a pivotal role. While the fundamental principles of macronutrients and micronutrients discussed in the previous chapter provide a solid foundation for an age-defying nutrition plan, there is a select group of nutrient-dense superfoods that stand out as particularly powerful allies in the fight against the ravages of time.

These anti-aging superfoods are not only packed with essential vitamins, minerals, and antioxidants, but they also possess unique bioactive compounds that can actively combat the underlying mechanisms of aging, from cellular inflammation to oxidative stress. By strategically incorporating these longevity-boosting superfoods into your daily diet, you can harness the power of nature to support optimal health, enhance your body's regenerative capacities, and defy the conventional wisdom of growing old.

Berries: The Antioxidant Powerhouses

Berries, with their vibrant colors and bursting flavors, are true nutritional superstars in the world of anti-aging superfoods. From blueberries and raspberries to acai and goji berries, these tiny fruits are brimming with a diverse array of polyphenolic compounds, potent antioxidants that can help neutralize harmful free radicals and reduce inflammation throughout the body.

Blueberries, for instance, are renowned for their high concentrations of anthocyanins, which have been shown to improve cognitive function, enhance memory, and even protect against age-related neurodegenerative conditions, such as Alzheimer's disease. These antioxidant-rich berries have also been linked to improved cardiovascular health, reduced risk of type 2 diabetes, and a stronger immune system – all of which are crucial for maintaining a vibrant, youthful life.

Raspberries, on the other hand, are a rich source of ellagitannins, a unique class of polyphenols that have been studied for their anti-cancer properties and their ability to support healthy aging. These berries are also a excellent source of fiber, which can promote gut health and regularity – both of which are essential for optimal nutrient absorption and overall well-being.

Exotic superfoods like acai and goji berries have also gained popularity in recent years for their exceptional antioxidant profiles and potential health benefits. Acai berries, for example, are brimming with anthocyanins and omega-fatty acids that can help reduce inflammation, support heart health, and even aid in weight management. Goji berries, on the other hand, are a rich source of carotenoids, such as zeaxanthin and lutein, which are essential for maintaining healthy vision and supporting the body's natural detoxification processes.

By incorporating a diverse array of berries into your daily diet, whether through fresh fruit, smoothies, or even unsweetened dried varieties, you can tap into the powerful anti-aging properties of these nutrient-dense superfoods and fortify your body's natural defenses against the ravages of time.

Leafy Greens: The Longevity Elixir

Leafy green vegetables, such as kale, spinach, and Swiss chard, are undoubtedly among the most potent anti-aging superfoods in the plant kingdom. These nutrient-dense powerhouses are brimming with a vast array of vitamins, minerals, and antioxidants that can help combat the underlying drivers of aging, from oxidative stress to chronic inflammation.

Kale, for instance, is a veritable treasure trove of longevity-boosting nutrients. This leafy green is an excellent source of vitamin K, which is essential for maintaining strong, healthy bones and reducing the risk of age-related osteoporosis. Kale is also rich in vitamin C, a powerful antioxidant that can help support the immune system, promote collagen production, and even improve the appearance of skin.

Spinach, another nutrient-dense superfood, is brimming with lutein and zeaxanthin – two carotenoids that have been shown to support eye health and protect against age-related macular degeneration, a leading cause of vision loss among older adults. Spinach is also a rich source of folate, a B vitamin that plays a crucial role in cellular repair and the production of DNA, both of which are essential for maintaining a youthful, vibrant body.

Swiss chard, with its striking rainbow of colors, is a nutritional powerhouse that boasts an impressive array of beneficial plant compounds, including betalains, which have been studied for their anti-inflammatory and antioxidant properties. This leafy green is also an excellent source of magnesium, a mineral that is essential for maintaining healthy blood pressure, supporting muscle and nerve function, and even regulating mood and cognitive abilities.

By incorporating a diverse array of leafy greens into your daily diet, you can create a symphony of longevity-boosting nutrients that can help fortify your body's natural defenses, combat the ravages of time, and unlock a new level of vibrant, youthful health.

Cruciferous Vegetables: The Cancer-Fighting Powerhouses

Cruciferous vegetables, such as broccoli, cauliflower, and Brussels sprouts, are a standout group of anti-aging superfoods that deserve special attention. These nutrient-dense veggies are not only packed with essential vitamins and minerals but also possess unique bioactive compounds that can actively combat the development of age-related diseases, particularly certain types of cancer.

At the heart of the cruciferous vegetable's anti-aging prowess lie compounds known as glucosinolates, which are broken down into biologically active substances, such as sulforaphane and indole-3-carbinol. These plant-based compounds have been extensively studied for their ability to inhibit the growth of cancer cells, reduce inflammation, and even support detoxification pathways within the body.

Broccoli, for instance, is a rich source of sulforaphane, a compound that has been shown to possess potent antioxidant and anti-inflammatory properties. Studies have linked the regular consumption of broccoli to a reduced risk of various types of cancer, including prostate, breast, and colon cancer – all of which become more prevalent with age.

Cauliflower, on the other hand, is a cruciferous vegetable that contains high levels of indole-3-carbinol, a compound that can help regulate estrogen metabolism and support hormonal balance – both of which are crucial for maintaining overall health and vitality as we grow older.

Brussels sprouts are another cruciferous superstar, brimming with a diverse array of beneficial plant compounds, including kaempferol and quercetin, which have been studied for their ability to protect against age-related cognitive decline and support cardiovascular health.

By incorporating a variety of cruciferous vegetables into your daily diet, you can harness the power of these nutrient-dense superfoods to combat the development of age-related diseases, support detoxification, and fortify your body's natural defenses against the ravages of time.

Fatty Fish: The Longevity Elixir of the Sea

While the benefits of plant-based superfoods are undeniable, the marine world also offers a treasure trove of anti-aging superstars in the form of fatty fish, such as salmon, sardines, and mackerel.

These oily fish are rich in long-chain omega-3 fatty acids, including eicosapentaenoic acid (EPA) and docosahexaenoic acid (DHA), which have been extensively studied for their profound impact on human health and longevity.

Omega-3 fatty acids are renowned for their potent anti-inflammatory properties, which can help combat the chronic inflammation that is often associated with the aging process. By reducing inflammation throughout the body, these healthy fats can help mitigate the risk of age-related diseases, such as heart disease, Alzheimer's, and certain types of cancer.

Moreover, the omega-3s found in fatty fish have been shown to support brain health and cognitive function, making them an essential component of an age-defying nutrition plan. DHA, in particular, is a critical structural component of the brain and has been linked to improved memory, enhanced focus, and a reduced risk of age-related cognitive decline.

Salmon, a true superfood of the sea, is an excellent source of both EPA and DHA, as well as a host of other longevity-boosting nutrients, including vitamin D, selenium, and astaxanthin – a powerful carotenoid antioxidant that can help protect the skin from the damaging effects of UV radiation.

Sardines, on the other hand, are a small but mighty superfood that are packed with omega-3s, vitamin B12, and calcium – all of which are essential for maintaining strong, healthy bones and supporting overall vitality as we age.

By incorporating fatty fish into your weekly meal rotation, you can reap the myriad benefits of these marine superfoods and fortify your body's defenses against the ravages of time. Whether you enjoy grilled salmon, baked mackerel, or a refreshing sardine salad, these nutrient-dense options can become powerful allies in your quest for vibrant, youthful health.

Nuts and Seeds: The Longevity Powerhouses

In the realm of anti-aging superfoods, nuts and seeds deserve a place of honor for their impressive nutritional profiles and their ability to support various aspects of healthy aging.

Almonds, for instance, are a rich source of vitamin E, a fat-soluble antioxidant that can help protect cells from oxidative damage and support a healthy immune system. These versatile nuts are also brimming with magnesium, a mineral that plays a crucial role in energy production, muscle function, and the regulation of blood pressure – all of which are essential for maintaining a vibrant, youthful life.

Walnuts, on the other hand, are renowned for their high content of alpha-linolenic acid (ALA), a plant-based omega-3 fatty acid that can help reduce inflammation, improve brain function, and even support heart health. These nutrient-dense nuts are also a excellent source of copper, a mineral that is essential for the production of collagen and the maintenance of healthy skin, joints, and blood vessels.

Chia seeds and flaxseeds are two other anti-aging superstars that deserve special attention. These tiny powerhouses are rich in omega-3 fatty acids, fiber, and a diverse array of antioxidants, making them a potent ally in the fight against the ravages of time. Chia seeds, for example, are brimming with calcium, which is crucial for maintaining strong, healthy bones, while flaxseeds are a excellent source of lignans, plant-based compounds that have been studied for their potential to reduce the risk of certain types of cancer.

By incorporating a variety of nutrient-dense nuts and seeds into your daily diet, whether through trail mixes, smoothies, or as a crunchy topping on salads and yogurt, you can tap into the longevity-boosting properties of these anti-aging superfoods and fortify your body's natural defenses against the passage of time.

The Synergistic Power of Anti-Aging Superfoods

While the individual anti-aging superfoods discussed in this chapter possess remarkable health-promoting properties, it is the synergistic interplay between them that truly unlocks the transformative potential of an age-defying nutrition plan.

By strategically combining a diverse array of these nutrient-dense power-houses, you can create a symphony of nourishment that supports the body's natural regenerative processes, reduces inflammation, and promotes overall well-being.

For instance, starting your day with a smoothie that features a blend of berries, leafy greens, and chia seeds can provide a powerful antioxidant boost, support cognitive function, and even aid in digestion and regularity – all of which are crucial for maintaining vibrant health as you age.

Pairing grilled salmon, a rich source of omega-3s, with a side of roasted broccoli, a cruciferous superfood brimming with cancer-fighting compounds, can help combat inflammation, support heart health, and fortify the body's natural defenses against age-related diseases.

Snacking on a handful of almonds and walnuts, combined with a serving of fresh fruit, such as blueberries or goji berries, can deliver a potent dose of longevity-boosting vitamins, minerals, and healthy fats that can help regulate blood sugar, enhance cognitive function, and promote overall well-being.

By embracing the collective power of these anti-aging superfoods and incorporating them into your daily diet, you can create a synergistic symphony of nourishment that can help you defy the limitations of time and reclaim your birthright to a life of vibrant, youthful health.

In the chapters that follow, we will explore practical strategies for seamlessly integrating these age-defying superfoods into your daily routine, as well as delve deeper into the specific health benefits and science-backed mechanisms behind their longevity-boosting properties. Get ready to embark on a culinary adventure that will transform the way you approach the aging process and unlock a new level of vitality and well-being.

# CHAPTER 3

Chapter 3: Gut Health and Longevity: The Gut-Brain Connection

As we delve deeper into the realm of age-defying nutrition, it's becoming increasingly clear that the key to unlocking vibrant, youthful health extends far beyond the food we consume. In fact, one of the most important, yet often overlooked, aspects of longevity is the health and balance of our gut microbiome – the trillions of microorganisms that reside within our digestive system.

The gut-brain connection is a fascinating and rapidly evolving area of scientific research, revealing the profound impact that our gut health can have on the aging process and our overall well-being. By understanding the intricate interplay between the gut and the brain, and the crucial role that gut microbiome plays in this dynamic relationship, we can unlock a powerful new dimension of an age-defying nutrition plan.

The Gut Microbiome: A Diverse Ecosystem of Longevity

The gut microbiome is a complex and diverse ecosystem, home to trillions of bacteria, viruses, fungi, and other microorganisms that play a vital role in our physical and mental health. This intricate community of microbes, often referred to as the "second brain," is essential for a wide range of physiological functions, from nutrient absorption and energy production to immune system regulation and hormone balance.

As we age, the composition and diversity of our gut microbiome can undergo significant changes, often leading to an imbalance or dysbiosis. This disruption in the delicate microbial equilibrium can have far-reaching consequences on our overall health, contributing to the development of age-related diseases, such as obesity, type 2 diabetes, cardiovascular disease, and cognitive decline.

Maintaining a healthy, diverse gut microbiome, therefore, is a crucial component of an age-defying nutrition plan. By nourishing the beneficial bacteria that reside within our digestive system, we can support the body's natural regenerative processes, combat inflammation, and promote a state of dynamic equilibrium that can help us defy the limitations of time.

The Gut-Brain Axis: The Bidirectional Superhighway
At the heart of the gut-health and longevity connection lies the intricate gut-brain axis – a complex, two-way communication network that links the gastrointestinal tract to the central nervous system. This bidirectional super-highway allows the gut and the brain to constantly exchange information, influencing each other's function and ultimately shaping our overall health and well-being.

The gut-brain axis is facilitated by a variety of neurological, hormonal, and immunological pathways, with the gut microbiome playing a pivotal role in this dynamic interplay. The microbes that reside within our digestive system produce a wide range of metabolites, neurotransmitters, and inflammatory mediators that can directly impact the function and structure of the brain.

For instance, the gut bacteria are responsible for the production of essential neurotransmitters, such as serotonin and gamma-aminobutyric acid (GABA), which are critical for regulating mood, cognition, and even sleep patterns. Imbalances in these neurotransmitters can contribute to the development of age-related mental health conditions, such as depression, anxiety, and dementia.

Moreover, the gut microbiome also plays a crucial role in the body's inflammatory response, producing both pro-inflammatory and anti-inflammatory compounds that can have a direct impact on the brain. Chronic inflammation, which is often associated with the aging process, has been linked to a host of neurological and cognitive issues, including cognitive decline, Alzheimer's disease, and Parkinson's disease.

By maintaining a healthy, diverse gut microbiome through strategic dietary and lifestyle choices, we can help strengthen the gut-brain axis, reducing inflammation, supporting neurotransmitter balance, and promoting optimal brain function – all of which are essential for preserving cognitive abilities and mental well-being as we age.

Prebiotics, Probiotics, and Fermented Foods: The Gut-Boosting Trifecta

In the quest for a vibrant, youthful life, the importance of nurturing a healthy gut microbiome cannot be overstated. To achieve this, we must focus on three key components: prebiotics, probiotics, and fermented foods.

Prebiotics: The Gut's Nutritional Fuel

Prebiotics are a special class of dietary fibers that serve as food for the beneficial bacteria in our gut. These indigestible carbohydrates, found in a variety of plant-based foods, help to nourish and support the growth of probiotics, enabling them to thrive and maintain a healthy balance within the gut.

Onions, garlic, bananas, and whole grains are all excellent sources of prebiotics, providing the gut microbiome with the necessary fuel to perform its vital functions. By incorporating these prebiotic-rich foods into your daily diet, you can create a hospitable environment for the beneficial bacteria to flourish, ultimately supporting overall gut health and promoting longevity.

Probiotics: The Gut's Microbial Allies

Probiotics are the live, beneficial bacteria and yeasts that reside within the gut, playing a crucial role in maintaining a healthy, balanced microbiome. These gut-friendly microorganisms can help improve nutrient absorption, regulate immune function, and even produce essential vitamins and metabolites that support overall health and well-being.

Fermented foods, such as yogurt, kefir, sauerkraut, and kimchi, are excellent sources of probiotics, as the fermentation process helps to cultivate and preserve these beneficial microbes. Introducing a variety of probiotic-rich foods into your diet can help replenish and diversify the gut microbiome, ultimately supporting digestive function, reducing inflammation, and promoting longevity.

Fermented Foods: The Gut's Microbial Powerhouses

Fermented foods, in addition to being a rich source of probiotics, also contain a wealth of beneficial compounds that can further support gut health and longevity. During the fermentation process, the microorganisms present in these foods produce a variety of bioactive substances, including enzymes, organic acids, and antioxidants, that can positively impact the gut microbiome and the body as a whole.

Sauerkraut, for instance, is a fermented cabbage dish that is brimming with lactic acid bacteria, which can help improve digestive function, enhance the absorption of nutrients, and even support the immune system. Likewise, kimchi, a traditional Korean fermented vegetable dish, is packed with a diverse array of beneficial microbes and antioxidants that can help combat inflammation and support overall health.

By incorporating a variety of prebiotic-rich, probiotic-packed, and fermented foods into your daily diet, you can create a synergistic gut-boosting plan that nourishes the beneficial bacteria in your digestive system, strengthens the gut-brain axis, and unlocks the secrets to vibrant, youthful health.

The Gut Microbiome and Longevity: The Scientific Evidence

The growing body of scientific research on the gut microbiome and its connection to longevity is nothing short of remarkable. Studies have consistently shown that the diversity and composition of the gut microbial community play a crucial role in various aspects of the aging process, from metabolic health and immune function to cognitive abilities and disease risk.

One comprehensive review, published in the journal Frontiers in Genetics, examined the impact of gut dysbiosis (an imbalance in the gut microbiome) on the hallmarks of aging, including cellular senescence, stem cell exhaustion, and altered intercellular communication. The researchers found that disruptions in the gut microbiome can contribute to the development of age-related diseases, such as type 2 diabetes, cardiovascular disease, and neurodegenerative disorders.

Another study, published in the journal Nature Metabolism, explored the link between the gut microbiome and longevity in a mouse model. The researchers discovered that the transfer of gut microbiota from young, healthy mice to old mice resulted in improved metabolic function, reduced inflammation, and even extended lifespan – a testament to the profound influence that the gut microbiome can have on the aging process.

Furthermore, a growing body of research has highlighted the role of the gut-brain axis in cognitive function and neurodegenerative diseases. A study published in the journal Frontiers in Aging Neuroscience found that the gut microbiome is intimately linked to the development of Alzheimer's disease, with imbalances in the microbial community contributing to neuroinflammation and impaired brain function.

By nurturing a healthy, diverse gut microbiome through strategic dietary and lifestyle choices, we can harness the power of the gut-brain connection to support cognitive abilities, reduce inflammation, and promote overall longevity. This holistic approach to gut health and aging is a crucial component of an age-defying nutrition plan, empowering us to take control of our destiny and defy the limitations of time.

## Cultivating a Gut-Friendly Lifestyle

Maintaining a vibrant, youthful life requires a multifaceted approach that goes beyond simply optimizing our dietary choices. To truly unlock the longevity-boosting potential of the gut microbiome, we must also consider the various lifestyle factors that can impact the delicate balance of our digestive ecosystem.

## Exercise: A Gut-Boosting Ally

Regular physical activity has been shown to play a crucial role in supporting a healthy gut microbiome. By engaging in a variety of exercise modalities, from cardiovascular workouts to strength training, you can help stimulate the growth and diversity of beneficial gut bacteria, ultimately reducing inflammation and promoting overall well-being.

The mechanism behind this gut-boosting effect of exercise is multifaceted, ranging from improved blood flow and nutrient delivery to the gut, to the modulation of the body's stress response and immune system. Additionally, exercise can help promote the production of short-chain fatty acids, which are essential for maintaining a healthy intestinal lining and supporting the growth of probiotic bacteria.

## Stress Management: A Gut-Soothing Imperative

Chronic stress is a well-known contributor to gut dysbiosis, as it can disrupt the delicate balance of the gut microbiome and promote the growth of harmful, inflammation-inducing bacteria. By incorporating effective stress management techniques into your daily routine, you can help mitigate the negative impact of stress on your gut health and support the overall longevity of your body and mind.

Practices such as meditation, deep breathing exercises, and mindfulness-based activities can help reduce the physiological and psychological responses to stress, ultimately promoting a healthier gut microbiome and supporting the gut-brain axis. Additionally, engaging in activities that bring you joy and a sense of purpose can also have a positive impact on your gut health and overall well-being.

Sleep: The Gut's Restorative Companion
The importance of quality sleep in maintaining a healthy gut microbiome cannot be overstated. During the restorative phases of sleep, the body undergoes a series of physiological processes that are essential for supporting the growth and diversity of beneficial gut bacteria.

Studies have shown that sleep deprivation or disruption can lead to significant changes in the gut microbial community, contributing to inflammation, metabolic dysregulation, and an increased risk of age-related diseases. By prioritizing quality sleep and practicing good sleep hygiene, you can help promote a thriving gut microbiome and unlock the longevity-boosting benefits of this vital connection.

By integrating these gut-friendly lifestyle practices into your daily routine, in conjunction with a nutrient-dense, age-defying diet, you can create a comprehensive plan that nourishes the gut microbiome, strengthens the gut-brain axis, and empowers you to defy the limitations of time.

As we continue our journey through the transformative world of longevity nutrition, the role of the gut microbiome will undoubtedly remain a central focus. By understanding the intricate interplay between the gut and the brain, and the profound impact that a healthy, diverse microbial community can have on our overall well-being, we can unlock the keys to vibrant, youthful health and reclaim our birthright to a life of boundless vitality.

# CHAPTER 4

Chapter 4: Hydration for Youthful Vitality

In the pursuit of vibrant, age-defying health, the importance of proper hydration often takes a backseat to the more glamorous aspects of nutrition and lifestyle. However, the truth is that water, the very foundation of life, plays a pivotal role in maintaining youthful vitality and combating the ravages of time.

As we age, our bodies undergo a gradual decline in their ability to regulate fluid balance, leading to a host of age-related issues, from dry skin and joint pain to cognitive decline and increased susceptibility to chronic diseases. By prioritizing optimal hydration as a core component of our age-defying nutrition plan, we can unlock a powerful ally in the fight against the aging process and reclaim our birthright to a life of boundless energy and vibrant health.

The Aging Body's Thirst for Water

Water is the most abundant substance in the human body, comprising up to 60% of our total body weight. This essential fluid serves as the foundation for countless physiological processes, from cellular function and waste removal to temperature regulation and nutrient transport.

As we age, however, our bodies undergo a gradual decline in their ability to maintain proper hydration. This is due, in part, to a decrease in total body water content, as well as a reduction in the efficiency of the body's thirst and fluid regulation mechanisms.

Older adults, in particular, often experience a diminished thirst response, making it more challenging to recognize the early signs of dehydration. This can lead to a cascading effect, where the body's tissues and organs become progressively dehydrated, contributing to a host of age-related problems, such as:

1. Skin Health: Dehydration can lead to the loss of skin elasticity and the development of wrinkles, as the skin's natural moisture barrier becomes compromised.

2. Joint Health: Adequate hydration is essential for maintaining the integrity of joint cartilage and synovial fluid, which helps to cushion and lubricate our joints. Dehydration can exacerbate age-related joint pain and stiffness.

3. Cognitive Function: The brain is highly dependent on proper hydration, as water is essential for maintaining neuronal function, neurotransmitter balance, and the efficient flow of oxygen and nutrients. Dehydration has been linked to impaired cognitive abilities, including memory, concentration, and decision-making.

4. Cardiovascular Health: Dehydration can strain the cardiovascular system, leading to an increased risk of high blood pressure, heart disease, and other age-related cardiovascular problems.

5. Kidney and Bladder Function: The kidneys and bladder rely on adequate hydration to effectively filter waste, regulate fluid balance, and maintain urinary tract health. Dehydration can contribute to the development of kidney stones and urinary tract infections, both of which become more common with age.

By recognizing the profound impact that hydration has on our overall health and well-being, we can take proactive steps to ensure that our bodies remain optimally hydrated throughout the aging process, unlocking a powerful ally in the fight against the ravages of time.

The Science of Hydration and Longevity

The scientific evidence surrounding the connection between hydration and longevity is both compelling and multifaceted. Numerous studies have explored the various ways in which proper hydration can support healthy aging and reduce the risk of age-related diseases.

One comprehensive review, published in the journal Nutrients, examined the role of hydration in the aging process, focusing on its impact on cellular function, cognitive abilities, and chronic disease risk. The researchers found that adequate hydration can help maintain cellular integrity, reduce oxidative stress, and support the body's natural detoxification processes – all of which are crucial for combating the underlying drivers of aging.

Another study, published in the European Journal of Nutrition, investigated the relationship between hydration status and cognitive function in older adults. The researchers discovered that individuals with higher levels of hydration exhibited better performance on a range of cognitive tests, including memory, attention, and processing speed. This finding highlights the vital role that water plays in supporting brain health and preserving mental acuity as we age.

Furthermore, a growing body of research has linked proper hydration to a reduced risk of chronic diseases, such as type 2 diabetes, cardiovascular disease, and certain types of cancer. A study published in the Journal of the American College of Nutrition, for instance, found that individuals who maintained optimal hydration levels had a lower risk of developing type 2 diabetes, underscoring the importance of water in regulating metabolic function and supporting overall health.

By harnessing the power of hydration and incorporating it into our age-defying nutrition plan, we can unlock a potent tool for combating the underlying drivers of aging, from cellular dysfunction to chronic inflammation. This holistic approach to longevity empowers us to take control of our destiny and reclaim our birthright to a life of vibrant, youthful vitality.

## The Age-Defying Benefits of Optimal Hydration

As we delve deeper into the science of hydration and longevity, it becomes increasingly clear that maintaining proper fluid balance is essential for unlocking a wide range of age-defying benefits. From supporting skin health and joint function to enhancing cognitive abilities and reducing the risk of chronic diseases, the far-reaching impact of optimal hydration is truly remarkable.

## Skin Health: Plump, Glowing, and Youthful

Adequate hydration is a key component of maintaining healthy, vibrant skin as we age. Water plays a crucial role in maintaining the skin's natural moisture barrier, which helps to prevent the loss of essential oils and nutrients, and retain the skin's elasticity and suppleness.

Dehydration, on the other hand, can lead to the acceleration of wrinkle formation, sagging, and age spots, as the skin's natural ability to repair and regenerate becomes compromised. By ensuring that our bodies are properly hydrated, we can help combat the visible signs of aging, promote a healthy, glowing complexion, and reclaim our youthful radiance.

## Joint Health: Lubrication and Cushioning for Mobility

Water is an essential component of the synovial fluid that lubricates and cushions our joints, helping to reduce friction and facilitate smooth, pain-free movement. As we age, the body's ability to produce and maintain this vital joint fluid can diminish, leading to the development of osteoarthritis and other age-related joint problems.

By staying hydrated, we can help support the integrity of our joint cartilage, reduce inflammation, and maintain the flexibility and range of motion needed to enjoy an active, vibrant lifestyle well into our golden years. This, in turn, can help prevent the onset of debilitating joint pain and stiffness, empowering us to move through the world with ease and confidence.

Cognitive Function: Hydration for a Sharp, Agile Mind

The brain, being one of the most metabolically active organs in the body, is highly dependent on proper hydration for optimal function. Water plays a crucial role in maintaining the delicate balance of neurotransmitters, regulating blood flow to the brain, and facilitating the efficient transport of oxygen and nutrients.

Dehydration, even at relatively mild levels, has been shown to impair cognitive abilities, such as memory, concentration, and decision-making. This is particularly concerning as we age, as the brain's vulnerability to the effects of dehydration can increase, contributing to the risk of age-related cognitive decline and neurodegenerative diseases.

By prioritizing optimal hydration as part of our age-defying nutrition plan, we can help support the brain's natural regenerative processes, enhance mental clarity and focus, and maintain a sharp, agile mind well into our later years.

Cardiovascular Health: Hydration for a Strong, Resilient Heart

The cardiovascular system is another essential component of the body that relies on proper hydration for optimal function. Water plays a critical role in regulating blood volume, blood pressure, and the efficient delivery of oxygen and nutrients to the body's cells and tissues.

Dehydration, on the other hand, can place undue strain on the cardiovascular system, leading to an increased risk of high blood pressure, heart disease, and other age-related cardiovascular problems. By maintaining adequate hydration, we can help support the heart's natural resilience, improve circulation, and reduce the likelihood of developing these potentially life-threatening conditions.

Kidney and Bladder Health: Hydration for Efficient Filtration and Elimination

The kidneys and bladder are the body's primary filtration and elimination systems, and they are highly dependent on proper hydration to function effectively. Water helps to flush out toxins and waste products, prevent the formation of kidney stones, and maintain urinary tract health.

As we age, the kidneys and bladder can become more vulnerable to the effects of dehydration, leading to an increased risk of urinary tract infections, incontinence, and other age-related urological problems. By prioritizing optimal hydration, we can help support the body's natural detoxification processes, reduce the burden on the kidneys and bladder, and maintain the overall health and function of these vital organs.

Harnessing the Power of Hydration: Strategies for Youthful Vitality

Now that we've explored the profound impact that proper hydration can have on various aspects of health and longevity, it's time to dive into the practical strategies for incorporating optimal hydration into our age-defying nutrition plan.

1. Drink Enough Water: The Recommended Daily Intake

The recommended daily water intake can vary depending on factors such as age, gender, activity level, and overall health status. As a general guideline, the National Academies of Sciences, Engineering, and Medicine recommend that adults consume approximately 15.5 cups (3.7 liters) of fluids per day for men and 11.5 cups (2.7 liters) for women.

However, it's important to note that these are general recommendations, and individual needs may vary. Factors such as climate, health conditions, and physical activity levels can all influence the amount of water required to maintain optimal hydration.

2. Diversify Your Fluid Intake: The Power of Hydrating Foods

While water is undoubtedly the foundation of optimal hydration, it's not the only fluid that can contribute to our overall fluid balance. Many fruits and vegetables, as well as herbal teas and infusions, can also be excellent sources of hydration.

For instance, watermelon, cucumber, and tomatoes are all water-rich foods that can help boost your fluid intake while also providing a host of beneficial nutrients. Herbal teas, such as chamomile, peppermint, and hibiscus, can also serve as delicious and hydrating alternatives to plain water.

By diversifying our fluid intake and incorporating a variety of hydrating foods and beverages into our daily routine, we can enhance the overall nutritional value of our age-defying plan while also supporting optimal hydration levels.

3. Customize Your Hydration: Individual Needs and Lifestyle Factors

It's important to remember that the optimal hydration level is not a one-size-fits-all solution. Each individual's needs may vary based on factors such as age, activity level, climate, and overall health status.

For example, individuals who live in hot or dry climates, or who engage in regular physical activity, may require a higher fluid intake to maintain proper hydration. Similarly, older adults may need to be more diligent in their hydration efforts, as the body's thirst mechanism can become less sensitive with age.

By tuning in to our body's unique needs and making adjustments to our hydration practices as necessary, we can ensure that we are consistently meeting our individual fluid requirements and unlocking the full spectrum of age-defying benefits that optimal hydration has to offer.

4. Hydration-Boosting Habits: Integrating Hydration into Your Lifestyle

Achieving optimal hydration is not just about drinking more water; it's about cultivating a lifestyle that supports and reinforces healthy hydration habits. By incorporating simple, yet effective, strategies into our daily routines, we can make hydration a seamless and effortless part of our age-defying journey.

Some examples of hydration-boosting habits include:
- Keeping a water bottle or glass of water within reach throughout the day
- Setting reminders or alarms to sip water regularly
- Incorporating hydrating foods and beverages into our meals and snacks
- Paying attention to the body's thirst cues and responding promptly
- Adjusting our hydration levels based on changes in activity, climate, or health status

By weaving these hydration-focused habits into the fabric of our daily lives, we can ensure that we are consistently meeting our fluid needs and unlocking the full spectrum of age-defying benefits that optimal hydration has to offer.

As we continue our journey towards vibrant, youthful health, the importance of proper hydration cannot be overstated. By prioritizing optimal fluid balance as a core component of our age-defying nutrition plan, we can fortify our bodies' natural defenses, support the regenerative processes that combat the ravages of time, and reclaim our birthright to a life of boundless energy and vitality.

# CHAPTER 5

Chapter 5: Intermittent Fasting: The Key to Cellular Rejuvenation

In the ever-evolving landscape of longevity and anti-aging strategies, one approach has emerged as a particularly powerful tool in our quest for vibrant, youthful health: intermittent fasting. This ancient practice, which involves cycling between periods of fasting and eating, has been the subject of extensive scientific research, revealing a compelling array of age-defying benefits that extend far beyond the realm of weight management.

As we delve into the transformative power of intermittent fasting, we will explore the underlying mechanisms that make this dietary strategy such a potent ally in the fight against the ravages of time. From the cellular-level processes of autophagy and stem cell regeneration to the systemic benefits of improved metabolic function and reduced inflammation, we will uncover the science-backed reasons why intermittent fasting should be a core component of any comprehensive age-defying nutrition plan.

The Science of Cellular Rejuvenation

At the heart of intermittent fasting's age-defying prowess lies its ability to stimulate a process known as autophagy – a crucial cellular recycling and renewal mechanism that plays a vital role in the fight against aging.

Autophagy is a natural, self-cleaning process in which the body's cells break down and recycle damaged or dysfunctional cellular components, such as proteins and organelles. This process not only helps to eliminate waste and toxins, but it also provides the building blocks for the creation of new, healthy cells – a vital component of maintaining cellular integrity and promoting longevity.

As we age, the body's natural autophagy processes can become impaired, leading to the accumulation of cellular debris and the gradual decline of cellular function. This, in turn, can contribute to the development of age-related diseases, such as neurodegenerative disorders, cardiovascular problems, and certain types of cancer.

Intermittent fasting, however, has been shown to be a powerful trigger for the induction of autophagy. During periods of fasting, the body enters a state of cellular stress, which activates a cascade of signaling pathways that stimulate the autophagy process. This cellular "housekeeping" allows the body to clear out damaged or dysfunctional components, making way for the regeneration of newer, healthier cells.

Furthermore, intermittent fasting has also been linked to the enhanced production of stem cells – the unspecialized cells that have the remarkable ability to differentiate into a wide variety of specialized cell types. By promoting the growth and proliferation of these regenerative stem cells, intermittent fasting can help the body replenish and rejuvenate damaged or aging tissues, supporting overall organ function and resilience.

The Metabolic Benefits of Intermittent Fasting

In addition to its profound impact on cellular processes, intermittent fasting has also been shown to offer a multitude of metabolic benefits that are essential for maintaining youthful vitality and combating the ravages of time.

One of the primary metabolic advantages of intermittent fasting is its ability to enhance insulin sensitivity and regulate blood sugar levels. As we age, the body's ability to effectively utilize insulin, the hormone responsible for regulating blood glucose, can become impaired, leading to the development of insulin resistance and an increased risk of type 2 diabetes.

Intermittent fasting, however, has been found to improve insulin sensitivity and help maintain healthy blood sugar levels, even in individuals with pre-existing metabolic conditions. This is achieved through a combination of mechanisms, including the reduction of inflammation, the enhancement of cellular energy production, and the optimization of hormonal signaling pathways.

By improving metabolic function and reducing the risk of insulin-related disorders, intermittent fasting can help prevent the cascade of age-related health issues that are often associated with metabolic dysfunction, such as cardiovascular disease, cognitive decline, and certain types of cancer.

Moreover, intermittent fasting has also been linked to the stimulation of a process known as "metabolic switching," where the body shifts from primarily using glucose as a fuel source to tapping into its fat reserves. This metabolic flexibility can not only support weight management and body composition but also enhance energy levels, cognitive function, and overall physical and mental performance – all of which are crucial for maintaining a vibrant, youthful lifestyle.

The Anti-Inflammatory Benefits of Intermittent Fasting

Chronic inflammation is widely recognized as a fundamental driver of the aging process, contributing to the development of a vast array of age-related diseases, from neurodegenerative disorders to cardiovascular problems. Fortunately, intermittent fasting has been shown to be a powerful tool in the fight against inflammation, offering a multifaceted approach to promoting overall health and longevity.

During periods of fasting, the body initiates a series of physiological responses that help to reduce inflammation at the cellular and systemic levels. For instance, intermittent fasting has been found to decrease the production of pro-inflammatory cytokines, while simultaneously enhancing the release of anti-inflammatory compounds, such as adiponectin and irisin.

Additionally, the cellular renewal and regeneration processes stimulated by intermittent fasting, such as autophagy and stem cell proliferation, can help to eliminate damaged or dysfunctional cells that may be contributing to the inflammatory response. This, in turn, can support the body's natural ability to maintain homeostasis and reduce the overall burden of inflammation.

Furthermore, the metabolic benefits of intermittent fasting, including improved insulin sensitivity and the optimization of energy production, can also play a crucial role in mitigating the inflammatory cascade. By regulating blood sugar levels, reducing oxidative stress, and enhancing mitochondrial function, intermittent fasting can help create an internal environment that is less conducive to the development and perpetuation of chronic inflammation.

By harnessing the anti-inflammatory power of intermittent fasting, we can help fortify our bodies' natural defenses against the ravages of time, reducing the risk of age-related diseases and supporting the maintenance of optimal health and vitality.

The Neurological and Cognitive Benefits of Intermittent Fasting

As we age, the health and resilience of our nervous system become increasingly crucial for maintaining cognitive abilities, emotional well-being, and overall quality of life. Fortunately, the benefits of intermittent fasting extend far beyond the realms of cellular renewal and metabolic optimization, reaching deep into the realm of neurological and cognitive function.

One of the primary ways in which intermittent fasting supports brain health is through its ability to stimulate the production of brain-derived neurotrophic factor (BDNF) – a crucial growth factor that plays a vital role in the creation of new neural connections, the survival of existing neurons, and the overall plasticity of the brain.

By enhancing BDNF levels, intermittent fasting can help improve memory, enhance learning, and support the brain's natural adaptive capacities – all of which are essential for combating age-related cognitive decline and preserving mental sharpness well into our golden years.

Moreover, the anti-inflammatory and metabolic benefits of intermittent fasting can also have a direct impact on neurological function. By reducing oxidative stress, improving insulin sensitivity, and promoting the efficient utilization of energy sources, intermittent fasting can help protect the brain from the deleterious effects of aging, including the development of neurodegenerative conditions, such as Alzheimer's and Parkinson's disease.

In addition to its neuroprotective effects, intermittent fasting has also been linked to improvements in mood and emotional well-being. The fasting-induced upregulation of neurotransmitters, such as serotonin and dopamine, can help alleviate symptoms of depression and anxiety, while also supporting overall psychological resilience and adaptability.

By integrating the powerful neurological and cognitive benefits of intermittent fasting into our age-defying nutrition plan, we can empower ourselves to maintain sharp, agile minds, robust emotional well-being, and a profound sense of mental clarity – all of which are essential for living a vibrant, youthful life.

Practical Strategies for Implementing Intermittent Fasting

Now that we've explored the science-backed benefits of intermittent fasting and its profound impact on cellular rejuvenation, metabolic function, and neurological health, it's time to dive into the practical strategies for incorporating this transformative dietary approach into our daily lives.

1. Choosing an Intermittent Fasting Protocol

One of the key advantages of intermittent fasting is its flexibility, as there are several different protocols and approaches that can be tailored to individual needs and preferences. Some of the most popular intermittent fasting methods include:

- Time-Restricted Eating (TRE): Limiting food consumption to a specific window of time, typically ranging from 8-12 hours, and fasting for the remaining hours of the day.

- 16:8 Fasting: Fasting for 16 hours and consuming all meals within an 8-hour window.

- 24-Hour Fasts: Fasting completely for 24 hours, 1-2 times per week.

- Alternate-Day Fasting: Cycling between a full fasting day and a day of normal eating.

The optimal intermittent fasting protocol will depend on your individual goals, lifestyle, and preferences. It's important to experiment and find the approach that fits seamlessly into your daily routine and supports your overall well-being.

2. Hydration and Nutrient-Dense Eating

During the fasting periods, it's crucial to maintain optimal hydration by drinking plenty of water, herbal teas, and other non-caloric beverages. This helps to support the body's natural detoxification processes and ensure that you are not confusing thirst for hunger.

When it comes to the eating windows, focus on nourishing your body with a balanced, nutrient-dense diet rich in whole, unprocessed foods. This includes a variety of vegetables, fruits, lean proteins, healthy fats, and complex carbohydrates – all of which will help to support the age-defying benefits of intermittent fasting.

3. Listening to Your Body and Making Adjustments

It's important to remember that the optimal intermittent fasting protocol may vary from person to person, and it may take some time and experimentation to find the approach that works best for you. Pay close attention to how your body responds to different fasting schedules and be prepared to make adjustments as needed.

Some individuals may thrive on a more aggressive fasting regimen, while others may prefer a more moderate approach. The key is to find the sweet spot that allows you to unlock the transformative benefits of intermittent fasting without compromising your overall health and well-being.

4. Incorporating Intermittent Fasting into Your Lifestyle

To truly harness the power of intermittent fasting and integrate it into a sustainable age-defying nutrition plan, it's essential to view this dietary approach as a lifestyle choice, rather than a temporary fix.

Incorporate intermittent fasting into your daily routine by planning your meals and fasting periods in advance, finding ways to stay hydrated and occupied during fasting windows, and gradually building up your tolerance and resilience over time.

Additionally, consider combining intermittent fasting with other age-defying practices, such as a nutrient-dense diet, regular exercise, and stress management techniques. By creating a holistic, synergistic approach to longevity, you can maximize the transformative benefits of intermittent fasting and unlock a new level of vibrant, youthful health.

As you embark on your intermittent fasting journey, remember to approach it with patience, flexibility, and a deep understanding of your body's unique needs. By doing so, you can tap into the profound cellular, metabolic, and neurological benefits of this transformative dietary strategy and reclaim your birthright to a life of boundless energy, sharp cognitive abilities, and vibrant, youthful vitality.

# CHAPTER 6

hapter 6: Exercise and Movement: Keeping Your Body Young

In the pursuit of vibrant, age-defying health, the role of exercise and movement cannot be overstated. While a nutrient-dense diet and strategic lifestyle practices, such as intermittent fasting, are essential components of an effective longevity plan, the synergistic power of physical activity is a crucial piece of the puzzle that unlocks the secrets to youthful vitality.

As we explore the transformative impact of exercise and movement on the aging process, we will delve into the science-backed mechanisms that make this age-old practice such a powerful ally in the fight against the ravages of time. From the cellular-level benefits of improved mitochondrial function and stem cell regeneration to the systemic advantages of enhanced cardiovascular health, metabolic optimization, and cognitive resilience, we will uncover the compelling reasons why regular physical activity should be a cornerstone of any comprehensive age-defying nutrition plan.

The Cellular Benefits of Exercise: Powering the Fountain of Youth

At the foundation of exercise's age-defying prowess lies its profound impact on cellular function and rejuvenation. As we age, our cells undergo a gradual decline in their ability to efficiently produce energy, repair damaged components, and maintain optimal homeostasis – all of which contribute to the hallmarks of the aging process, from cellular senescence to impaired tissue regeneration.

However, regular physical activity has been shown to catalyze a cascade of cellular-level processes that can help combat these age-related changes and support the body's natural regenerative capacities.

One of the primary ways in which exercise exerts its age-defying influence is through its ability to enhance mitochondrial function. Mitochondria, often referred to as the "powerhouses" of our cells, are responsible for the production of adenosine triphosphate (ATP), the primary currency of cellular energy. As we grow older, mitochondrial dysfunction can lead to a decline in energy production, increased oxidative stress, and the accelerated aging of our cells.

Exercise, however, has been found to stimulate the biogenesis and improved efficiency of mitochondria, enabling our cells to generate more ATP and operate at a higher level of metabolic function. This, in turn, can help combat the cellular hallmarks of aging, such as reduced protein synthesis, impaired DNA repair, and the accumulation of cellular waste and debris.

Moreover, exercise has also been linked to the induction of autophagy – the cellular "housekeeping" process that eliminates damaged or dysfunctional components and recycles their building blocks to create new, healthier cells. By promoting this crucial form of cellular renewal, exercise can help support the body's natural rejuvenation processes and combat the age-related decline in cellular integrity.

Furthermore, physical activity has been shown to stimulate the production and mobilization of stem cells – the undifferentiated cells that have the remarkable ability to transform into a wide variety of specialized cell types. This stem cell-boosting effect of exercise can help replenish and regenerate aging tissues, supporting the body's natural healing and repair mechanisms and maintaining optimal organ function as we grow older.

By harnessing the cellular-level benefits of exercise, we can fortify our bodies' natural defenses against the ravages of time, supporting the foundations of youthful vitality and unlocking a new level of vibrant health.

The Cardiovascular Benefits of Exercise: Promoting a Strong, Resilient Heart
As we age, the health and resilience of our cardiovascular system become increasingly crucial for maintaining overall well-being and longevity. Fortunately, exercise has been consistently shown to be a powerful ally in the fight against age-related cardiovascular decline, offering a multifaceted approach to supporting heart health and reducing the risk of life-threatening conditions.

One of the primary ways in which exercise benefits the cardiovascular system is through its ability to improve endothelial function – the health and responsiveness of the inner lining of our blood vessels. As we grow older, the endothelium can become less efficient at regulating blood flow, blood pressure, and the overall flexibility of our arteries, leading to an increased risk of hypertension, atherosclerosis, and other cardiovascular problems.

Regular physical activity, however, has been found to enhance endothelial function, promoting the production of nitric oxide and improving the blood vessels' ability to dilate and respond to changes in demand. This, in turn, can help lower blood pressure, improve circulation, and reduce the overall burden on the cardiovascular system.

Moreover, exercise has also been shown to play a crucial role in the maintenance of healthy cholesterol levels and the reduction of harmful triglycerides – two key factors in the prevention of heart disease and stroke. By encouraging the body to utilize fat as a fuel source and supporting the liver's ability to metabolize cholesterol, exercise can help keep our cardiovascular system running smoothly and efficiently as we age.

Furthermore, the positive impact of exercise on metabolic function, including enhanced insulin sensitivity and improved glucose regulation, can also have a profound effect on cardiovascular health. By helping to mitigate the risks associated with conditions like type 2 diabetes, which are often closely linked to age-related cardiovascular problems, exercise can serve as a powerful preventive measure against life-threatening heart-related issues.

By integrating regular physical activity into our age-defying nutrition plan, we can fortify the health and resilience of our cardiovascular system, reducing the risk of age-related heart disease and empowering ourselves to maintain a strong, vibrant heart well into our golden years.

The Metabolic Benefits of Exercise: Fueling Youthful Vitality

As we delve deeper into the age-defying benefits of exercise, it becomes clear that the positive impact extends far beyond the cardiovascular system, reaching deep into the realm of metabolic function – a crucial determinant of overall health and longevity.

One of the primary ways in which exercise supports metabolic well-being is through its ability to enhance insulin sensitivity and regulate blood sugar levels. As we age, the body's ability to effectively utilize insulin, the hormone responsible for managing blood glucose, can become impaired, leading to the development of insulin resistance and an increased risk of type 2 diabetes.

Regular physical activity, however, has been found to improve insulin sensitivity and help maintain healthy blood sugar levels, even in individuals with pre-existing metabolic conditions. This is achieved through a combination of mechanisms, including the stimulation of glucose uptake by muscle cells, the promotion of mitochondrial function, and the reduction of inflammation – all of which work together to optimize metabolic efficiency and support youthful vitality.

Moreover, exercise has also been shown to play a crucial role in the regulation of body composition, helping to maintain lean muscle mass and support healthy weight management – both of which are essential for combating the age-related decline in physical function and the increased risk of chronic diseases.

As we grow older, the natural tendency for muscle mass to diminish can contribute to a host of age-related problems, from reduced strength and mobility to an increased susceptibility to falls and fractures. However, regular physical activity, particularly strength training and resistance exercises, can help preserve and even build lean muscle, supporting overall physical function and resilience.

Additionally, the calorie-burning and fat-burning effects of exercise can help prevent the accumulation of excess body fat, which has been linked to a variety of age-related health issues, including cardiovascular disease, metabolic syndrome, and certain types of cancer.

By harnessing the metabolic benefits of exercise, we can fortify our bodies' natural defenses against the ravages of time, optimizing our energy production, regulating our weight, and maintaining the physical capabilities needed to live a vibrant, youthful life.

The Cognitive and Neurological Benefits of Exercise

As we age, the health and resilience of our nervous system become increasingly crucial for maintaining cognitive abilities, emotional well-being, and overall quality of life. Fortunately, the age-defying benefits of exercise extend far beyond the realms of cellular function and metabolic optimization, reaching deep into the realm of neurological and cognitive function.

One of the primary ways in which exercise supports brain health is through its ability to stimulate the production of brain-derived neurotrophic factor (BDNF) – a crucial growth factor that plays a vital role in the creation of new neural connections, the survival of existing neurons, and the overall plasticity of the brain.

By enhancing BDNF levels, exercise can help improve memory, enhance learning, and support the brain's natural adaptive capacities – all of which are essential for combating age-related cognitive decline and preserving mental sharpness well into our golden years.

Moreover, the positive impact of exercise on cardiovascular health and metabolic function can also have a direct influence on neurological function. By improving blood flow, reducing inflammation, and optimizing energy production, physical activity can help protect the brain from the deleterious effects of aging, including the development of neurodegenerative conditions, such as Alzheimer's and Parkinson's disease.

In addition to its neuroprotective effects, exercise has also been linked to improvements in mood and emotional well-being. The release of endorphins and the regulation of neurotransmitters, such as serotonin and dopamine, can help alleviate symptoms of depression and anxiety, while also supporting overall psychological resilience and adaptability.

By integrating the powerful cognitive and neurological benefits of exercise into our age-defying nutrition plan, we can empower ourselves to maintain sharp, agile minds, robust emotional well-being, and a profound sense of mental clarity – all of which are essential for living a vibrant, youthful life.

Practical Strategies for Incorporating Exercise and Movement

Now that we've explored the science-backed benefits of exercise and movement, it's time to dive into the practical strategies for integrating this transformative practice into our daily lives and unlocking its full age-defying potential.

1. Embrace a Diverse Fitness Regimen

To maximize the longevity-boosting benefits of exercise, it's important to incorporate a variety of movement modalities into your routine. This can include a combination of cardiovascular exercises, strength training, flexibility/mobility work, and even low-impact activities like walking, yoga, or Tai Chi.

By diversifying your physical activities, you can target different physiological systems, challenge your body in new ways, and ensure that you are supporting overall health and resilience as you age.

2. Prioritize Strength Training

As we grow older, the natural tendency for muscle mass to decline can have a profound impact on physical function, mobility, and the risk of age-related injuries. To combat this, it's essential to prioritize strength-based exercises, such as resistance training, weightlifting, or bodyweight exercises, as a core component of your fitness regimen.

Strength training not only helps preserve and even build lean muscle mass but also supports bone density, enhances metabolic function, and improves overall physical capabilities – all of which are crucial for maintaining youthful vitality.

3. Incorporate High-Intensity Interval Training (HIIT)

High-Intensity Interval Training (HIIT) has emerged as a highly effective exercise strategy for unlocking the age-defying benefits of physical activity. This form of training, which involves alternating short bursts of intense exercise with periods of rest or lower-intensity activity, has been shown to enhance mitochondrial function, improve cardiovascular health, and support metabolic optimization.

By incorporating HIIT workouts into your routine, you can maximize the cellular and physiological benefits of exercise, all while minimizing the time commitment – a valuable asset in our busy, modern lives.

4. Listen to Your Body and Make Adjustments

It's important to remember that the optimal exercise regimen may vary from person to person, and it may take some time and experimentation to find the approach that works best for you. Pay close attention to how your body responds to different fitness activities and be prepared to make adjustments as needed.

Some individuals may thrive on a more vigorous, high-intensity approach, while others may prefer a more gentle, low-impact routine. The key is to find the sweet spot that allows you to unlock the transformative benefits of exercise without compromising your overall health and well-being.

5. Incorporate Movement into Your Daily Routine

To truly harness the power of exercise and movement, it's essential to view it as a lifestyle choice, rather than a separate, scheduled activity. Look for opportunities to incorporate movement into your daily routine, whether it's taking regular walking breaks, choosing the stairs over the elevator, or engaging in light stretching or bodyweight exercises throughout the day.

By making physical activity a seamless and integral part of your daily life, you can create a sustainable, long-term approach to longevity that empowers you to maintain a vibrant, youthful lifestyle well into your golden years.

As you embark on your journey of exercise and movement, remember to approach it with patience, flexibility, and a deep understanding of your body's unique needs. By doing so, you can tap into the profound cellular, cardiovascular, metabolic, and neurological benefits of physical activity and reclaim your birthright to a life of boundless energy, sharp cognitive abilities, and vibrant, youthful vitality.

# CHAPTER 7

Chapter 7: Stress Management: Nurturing Your Mind-Body Connection

In the relentless pursuit of vibrant, age-defying health, the role of stress management cannot be overstated. While the foundations of our age-defying nutrition plan – a nutrient-dense diet, strategic exercise, and targeted longevity-boosting practices – are undoubtedly essential, the ability to effectively manage and mitigate the impact of stress is a crucial piece of the puzzle that can unlock the secrets to youthful vitality.

As we delve into the transformative power of stress management, we will explore the profound ways in which chronic stress can accelerate the aging process, contributing to a host of age-related health issues, from cellular dysfunction and metabolic dysregulation to cognitive decline and emotional well-being. Conversely, we will uncover the science-backed mechanisms by which mindfulness, relaxation techniques, and other stress-reducing practices can help us combat the ravages of time and reclaim our birthright to a life of boundless energy and resilience.

The Aging Impact of Chronic Stress

Stress, in its various forms – whether it be physical, emotional, or psychological – is a natural and unavoidable part of the human experience. However, when stress becomes chronic and unmanaged, it can have a devastating impact on our overall health and well-being, accelerating the aging process and increasing our susceptibility to a wide range of age-related diseases.

At the cellular level, chronic stress can contribute to the premature aging of our cells by triggering the shortening of telomeres – the protective caps at the ends of our chromosomes. Telomere length is closely associated with cellular lifespan, and the accelerated erosion of these crucial structures can lead to increased cellular senescence, impaired cellular function, and a heightened risk of age-related disorders.

Moreover, stress can also disrupt the delicate balance of our hormonal systems, leading to the overproduction of cortisol – the body's primary stress hormone. Elevated cortisol levels have been linked to a host of age-related problems, including increased abdominal fat, insulin resistance, and the suppression of the immune system – all of which can have far-reaching consequences on our overall health and longevity.

Chronic stress has also been shown to contribute to the development of systemic inflammation, a fundamental driver of the aging process. By triggering the release of pro-inflammatory cytokines and promoting the activation of inflammatory pathways, stress can fuel the progression of age-related diseases, such as cardiovascular problems, neurodegenerative disorders, and certain types of cancer.

Furthermore, the toll that stress takes on our mental and emotional well-being can also have a profound impact on our physical health and longevity. Conditions such as depression, anxiety, and burnout have all been associated with an increased risk of age-related cognitive decline, reduced immune function, and a lower overall quality of life.

By recognizing the pervasive and far-reaching influence of chronic stress on the aging process, we can begin to understand the critical importance of incorporating effective stress management strategies into our comprehensive age-defying nutrition plan. Only by nurturing the mind-body connection and fostering a state of resilience and equilibrium can we truly unlock the secrets to vibrant, youthful health.

The Science of Stress Management and Longevity

As we explore the science behind the age-defying benefits of stress management, it becomes clear that the mind-body connection is a powerful and multifaceted pathway to longevity. By engaging in a variety of relaxation techniques, mindfulness practices, and lifestyle interventions, we can harness the body's natural mechanisms for combating the ravages of time and supporting optimal health and well-being.

Mindfulness and Meditation: Cultivating Mental Resilience

At the heart of effective stress management lies the practice of mindfulness and meditation – techniques that have been shown to have a profound impact on both psychological and physiological well-being.

Mindfulness, the art of being fully present and attentive in the current moment, can help individuals develop a greater sense of self-awareness, emotional regulation, and the ability to respond to stressors with clarity and equanimity. By cultivating this state of heightened consciousness, we can break free from the cycle of rumination, worry, and reactivity that often characterizes the modern, fast-paced lifestyle – a critical step in fostering resilience and longevity.

The regular practice of meditation, in particular, has been extensively studied for its ability to positively influence the aging process. By inducing a state of deep relaxation and promoting the activation of the parasympathetic nervous system (the "rest and digest" response), meditation can help reduce the physiological effects of stress, including the production of cortisol and the perpetuation of inflammation.

Moreover, research has shown that regular meditation can actually induce structural and functional changes in the brain, including the thickening of the prefrontal cortex (associated with decision-making and emotional regulation) and the increased activation of regions involved in memory, learning, and emotional processing. These neuroplastic changes can help us maintain cognitive abilities, emotional well-being, and a heightened sense of presence as we grow older.

By incorporating mindfulness and meditation practices into our daily lives, we can cultivate a profound sense of mental and emotional resilience, empowering ourselves to navigate the challenges of aging with grace, clarity, and a renewed zest for life.

Breathwork and Relaxation Techniques: Optimizing Physiological Function
  Alongside the mental and emotional benefits of stress management, the strategic use of breathwork and relaxation techniques can also have a profound impact on our physical health and longevity.

Proper breathing, with its ability to influence the autonomic nervous system, can help regulate the body's stress response, reduce inflammation, and promote the efficient utilization of oxygen – all of which are crucial for maintaining optimal cellular function and supporting the body's natural regenerative processes.

Practices such as diaphragmatic breathing, box breathing, and Wim Hof method have all been studied for their potential to enhance mitochondrial function, boost the immune system, and even stimulate the release of endorphins – the body's natural feel-good chemicals that can help alleviate symptoms of depression and anxiety.

Furthermore, the incorporation of relaxation techniques, such as progressive muscle relaxation, guided imagery, and yoga, can also play a vital role in the management of stress and the promotion of longevity. By deliberately inducing a state of physical and mental relaxation, we can help the body return to a state of homeostasis, reducing the wear and tear of chronic stress and supporting the body's natural ability to heal, repair, and rejuvenate.

By harnessing the power of breathwork and relaxation techniques, we can fortify the mind-body connection, optimize physiological function, and unlock the secrets to vibrant, youthful health.

Lifestyle Interventions: Fostering a Stress-Resilient Lifestyle

While the incorporation of mindfulness practices and relaxation techniques is undoubtedly essential for effective stress management, the reality is that the journey to longevity must extend beyond these individual practices. To truly harness the age-defying benefits of stress reduction, we must also address the broader lifestyle factors that contribute to our overall well-being and resilience.

One of the key lifestyle interventions that can have a profound impact on stress management and longevity is the prioritization of quality sleep. Adequate, high-quality sleep is essential for the body's natural restorative processes, the regulation of hormones, and the maintenance of cognitive function – all of which are crucial for combating the ravages of time.

By establishing consistent sleep hygiene habits, such as maintaining a regular sleep-wake cycle, creating a soothing sleep environment, and limiting exposure to blue light before bedtime, we can help ensure that our bodies are able to enter the deep, restorative stages of sleep that are so essential for optimal health and longevity.

Additionally, the incorporation of social connection and community engagement can also play a vital role in the management of stress and the promotion of overall well-being. Numerous studies have shown that individuals with strong social support networks and a sense of belonging tend to experience lower levels of stress, reduced inflammation, and a greater overall sense of life satisfaction – all of which can contribute to increased longevity.

By fostering meaningful relationships, participating in social activities, and engaging in community-based initiatives, we can not only alleviate the burden of isolation and loneliness (common challenges faced by older adults) but also tap into the profound psychological and physiological benefits of social connectedness.

Furthermore, the integration of recreational and leisure activities into our daily lives can also serve as a powerful stress management tool. Whether it's indulging in a favorite hobby, immersing ourselves in nature, or engaging in creative pursuits, these "joyful" experiences can help us cultivate a greater sense of purpose, reduce the symptoms of burnout, and support overall emotional well-being – all of which are essential for maintaining vibrant, youthful health.

By adopting a holistic, lifestyle-based approach to stress management, we can create a comprehensive age-defying plan that empowers us to nurture the mind-body connection, foster resilience, and unlock the secrets to a life of boundless energy and vitality.

Integrating Stress Management into Your Age-Defying Nutrition Plan

Now that we've explored the profound impact of stress management on the aging process and the science-backed strategies for cultivating a stress-resilient lifestyle, it's time to delve into the practical steps for seamlessly integrating these transformative practices into our comprehensive age-defying nutrition plan.

1. Establish a Mindfulness and Meditation Practice

Commit to a regular mindfulness and meditation practice, even if it's just for a few minutes each day. Start with a simple breathing meditation or a guided mindfulness exercise, and gradually build up the duration and depth of your practice over time.

Remember, there is no one-size-fits-all approach to meditation and mindfulness – experiment with different techniques and find the ones that resonate most with you and your lifestyle. The key is to make it a consistent, sustainable habit that becomes an integral part of your daily routine.

2. Incorporate Breathwork and Relaxation Techniques

Alongside your mindfulness and meditation practice, make time to integrate breathwork and relaxation techniques into your daily life. This could include diaphragmatic breathing exercises, yoga sequences, or even simple body scans and progressive muscle relaxation.

By consciously allocating time for these restorative practices, you can help regulate your autonomic nervous system, reduce inflammation, and support the body's natural rejuvenation processes – all of which are crucial for maintaining vibrant, youthful health.

3. Prioritize Quality Sleep and Social Connectedness

Establish consistent sleep hygiene habits, such as maintaining a regular sleep-wake cycle, creating a soothing sleep environment, and limiting exposure to blue light before bedtime. Additionally, make a concerted effort to nurture your social connections, whether it's through regular meetups with friends, joining a community group, or engaging in volunteer work.

By prioritizing these lifestyle factors, you can help alleviate the burden of stress, support your emotional well-being, and unlock the profound longevity-boosting benefits of a well-rested, socially engaged mind and body.

4. Embrace Joyful Leisure Activities

Carve out time in your schedule for recreational and leisure activities that bring you a genuine sense of joy and fulfillment. Whether it's indulging in a creative hobby, immersing yourself in nature, or simply engaging in a favorite pastime, these "joyful" experiences can help reduce the symptoms of burnout, foster a greater sense of purpose, and support overall emotional well-being.

5. Tailor Your Stress Management Strategies to Your Unique Needs

Remember that the optimal stress management plan is not a one-size-fits-all solution. Pay close attention to how your body and mind respond to the different practices and interventions, and be prepared to make adjustments as needed.

Some individuals may thrive on a more rigorous, high-intensity approach to stress management, while others may prefer a more gentle, restorative routine. The key is to find the sweet spot that allows you to unlock the transformative benefits of stress reduction without compromising your overall health and well-being.

As you embark on your stress management journey, embrace an attitude of curiosity, self-compassion, and a willingness to experiment. By nurturing the mind-body connection and fostering a state of resilience and equilibrium, you can unlock the secrets to vibrant, youthful health and reclaim your birthright to a life of boundless energy, sharp cognitive abilities, and emotional well-being.

# CHAPTER 8

C hapter 8: Sleep and Rejuvenation: Unlocking the Fountain of Youth

In the pursuit of vibrant, age-defying health, the role of sleep often takes a backseat to the more glamorous aspects of nutrition and lifestyle. However, the truth is that quality sleep, the very foundation of our daily lives, plays a pivotal role in maintaining youthful vitality and combating the ravages of time.

As we age, our sleep patterns and the restorative processes that occur during slumber can undergo significant changes, leading to a host of age-related issues, from cognitive decline and hormonal imbalances to increased susceptibility to chronic diseases. By prioritizing optimal sleep as a core component of our age-defying nutrition plan, we can unlock a powerful ally in the fight against the aging process and reclaim our birthright to a life of boundless energy and rejuvenation.

The Aging Body's Changing Sleep Needs

Sleep is a fundamental physiological process that is essential for the maintenance of overall health and well-being. During the various stages of sleep, the body undergoes a series of restorative and regenerative processes, from the consolidation of memories and the regulation of hormones to the repair of cells and the strengthening of the immune system.

However, as we grow older, the body's sleep architecture and the underlying mechanisms that govern our sleep-wake cycles can undergo significant changes, often leading to a decline in the quality and quantity of sleep.

One of the primary age-related changes in sleep patterns is the decrease in the amount of time spent in deep, slow-wave sleep – the most restorative stage of the sleep cycle. As we age, the brain's ability to generate the slow, high-amplitude brain waves that characterize this stage of sleep can diminish, resulting in a reduction in the body's ability to perform crucial cellular repair and tissue regeneration processes.

Additionally, older adults often experience an increase in the frequency and duration of wakefulness during the night, a condition known as sleep fragmentation. This disruption in the continuity of sleep can lead to a host of problems, including daytime fatigue, cognitive impairment, and an increased risk of chronic health conditions.

Furthermore, the aging process can also impact the body's circadian rhythms – the internal biological clocks that regulate our sleep-wake cycles. As we grow older, the body's ability to maintain a consistent and well-synchronized circadian rhythm can become compromised, leading to issues such as delayed sleep onset, early-morning wakeups, and a general disruption in the natural ebb and flow of the sleep-wake cycle.

These age-related changes in sleep patterns and the underlying biological mechanisms that govern them can have far-reaching consequences on our overall health and well-being, contributing to a wide range of age-related problems, from cognitive decline and hormonal imbalances to an increased risk of chronic diseases, such as cardiovascular problems, metabolic disorders, and certain types of cancer.

The Science of Sleep and Longevity

The scientific evidence surrounding the connection between sleep and longevity is both compelling and multifaceted. Numerous studies have explored the various ways in which quality sleep can support healthy aging and reduce the risk of age-related diseases.

One comprehensive review, published in the journal Frontiers in Neuroscience, examined the impact of sleep on the hallmarks of aging, including cellular senescence, genomic instability, and epigenetic alterations. The researchers found that adequate, high-quality sleep can help mitigate the detrimental effects of these age-related changes, promoting cellular rejuvenation, preserving genomic integrity, and supporting overall physiological function.

Another study, published in the journal Sleep Medicine Reviews, investigated the relationship between sleep disturbances and the risk of developing neurodegenerative diseases. The researchers discovered that individuals with chronic sleep issues, such as sleep apnea and insomnia, exhibited a higher incidence of cognitive decline and an increased likelihood of developing conditions like Alzheimer's and Parkinson's disease.

Furthermore, a growing body of research has linked quality sleep to improved metabolic function, reduced inflammation, and a lower risk of chronic diseases, such as type 2 diabetes, cardiovascular problems, and certain types of cancer. A study published in the journal Sleep, for instance, found that individuals who consistently obtained sufficient, high-quality sleep had a reduced likelihood of developing metabolic syndrome – a cluster of conditions that can significantly increase the risk of age-related health issues.

By harnessing the power of sleep and incorporating it into our age-defying nutrition plan, we can unlock a potent tool for combating the underlying drivers of aging, from cellular dysfunction to chronic inflammation. This holistic approach to longevity empowers us to take control of our destiny and reclaim our birthright to a life of vibrant, youthful vitality.

The Age-Defying Benefits of Quality Sleep

As we delve deeper into the science of sleep and longevity, it becomes increasingly clear that maintaining optimal sleep quality and quantity is essential for unlocking a wide range of age-defying benefits. From supporting cellular regeneration and cognitive function to regulating hormonal balance and reducing the risk of chronic diseases, the far-reaching impact of quality sleep is truly remarkable.

Cellular Rejuvenation: The Fountain of Youth at Work

During the various stages of sleep, the body undergoes a series of restorative processes that are crucial for cellular health and longevity. One of the primary ways in which sleep supports cellular rejuvenation is through the process of autophagy – the cellular "housekeeping" mechanism that eliminates damaged or dysfunctional components and recycles their building blocks to create new, healthier cells.

Studies have shown that the deep, slow-wave sleep stage is particularly important for the induction of autophagy, as it is during this time that the body's energy resources are directed towards the repair and regeneration of cells. By maintaining adequate, high-quality sleep, we can help support this crucial cellular cleansing process, combating the accumulation of cellular waste and debris that can contribute to the aging process.

Moreover, sleep also plays a vital role in the regulation of telomeres – the protective caps at the ends of our chromosomes that are closely associated with cellular lifespan. Chronic sleep deprivation has been linked to the accelerated shortening of telomeres, which can lead to increased cellular senescence and an elevated risk of age-related diseases.

By prioritizing quality sleep as part of our age-defying nutrition plan, we can help support the body's natural cellular rejuvenation processes, fostering a state of dynamic equilibrium and unlocking the secrets to vibrant, youthful health.

Cognitive Function: Sharpening the Mind

As we age, the health and resilience of our cognitive abilities become increasingly crucial for maintaining a high quality of life and preserving our independence. Fortunately, quality sleep plays a pivotal role in supporting brain function and combating age-related cognitive decline.

During the various stages of sleep, the brain undergoes a series of crucial processes, including the consolidation of memories, the reorganization of neural connections, and the clearance of waste products. These restorative activities are essential for maintaining cognitive agility, preserving learning and memory capabilities, and supporting the overall health and adaptability of the brain.

Studies have consistently shown that individuals who obtain sufficient, high-quality sleep exhibit better performance on a range of cognitive tests, including measures of attention, problem-solving, and verbal fluency. Conversely, chronic sleep deprivation has been linked to an increased risk of age-related cognitive impairment, including the development of neurodegenerative conditions like Alzheimer's disease.

By ensuring that we are obtaining the recommended amount of sleep and prioritizing the maintenance of a consistent, well-synchronized sleep-wake cycle, we can help support the brain's natural regenerative processes and preserve our mental sharpness well into our golden years.

Hormonal Balance: The Key to Youthful Vitality

Sleep plays a crucial role in the regulation of the body's endocrine system, which is responsible for the production and distribution of hormones – the chemical messengers that govern a wide range of physiological processes, from metabolism and growth to sexual function and mood.

As we age, the body's ability to maintain hormonal balance can become compromised, leading to a variety of age-related issues, such as weight gain, sexual dysfunction, and mood disorders. Fortunately, quality sleep can help support the optimal functioning of the endocrine system, promoting the secretion of hormones that are essential for maintaining youthful vitality.

For instance, deep, slow-wave sleep is crucial for the production of growth hormone – a crucial anabolic hormone that plays a vital role in the maintenance of lean muscle mass, the regulation of body composition, and the support of the body's natural regenerative processes. Chronic sleep deprivation, on the other hand, can lead to a decrease in growth hormone secretion, contributing to the age-related decline in physical function and overall well-being.

Similarly, sleep also influences the body's production of melatonin – the "sleep hormone" that not only regulates the sleep-wake cycle but also possesses potent antioxidant properties and has been linked to the reduction of inflammation, a fundamental driver of the aging process.

By prioritizing quality sleep and maintaining a consistent sleep-wake rhythm, we can help support the body's natural hormonal balance, promoting youthful vitality, optimal metabolic function, and a heightened sense of overall well-being.

Immune Function: The Bodyguard Against Age-Related Diseases

The immune system, which is responsible for protecting the body against a wide range of threats, including infections, diseases, and cellular damage, plays a crucial role in the maintenance of health and longevity. Fortunately, quality sleep has been shown to be a powerful ally in supporting the immune system and reducing the risk of age-related diseases.

During the sleep cycle, the body undergoes a series of immune-boosting processes, including the increased production of cytokines – signaling molecules that help coordinate the immune response. These cytokines, along with other immune cells, are crucial for the body's ability to recognize and eliminate harmful pathogens, as well as to repair damaged tissues and support the regeneration of healthy cells.

Furthermore, sleep also plays a role in the regulation of inflammation, a double-edged sword that can contribute to the development of age-related diseases when left unchecked. By supporting the body's natural anti-inflammatory processes and helping to maintain a balanced inflammatory response, quality sleep can serve as a powerful defense against the ravages of chronic inflammation.

Conversely, chronic sleep deprivation has been linked to an increased risk of a wide range of age-related health problems, including cardiovascular disease, neurodegenerative disorders, and certain types of cancer. This is due, in part, to the negative impact that lack of sleep can have on the immune system, leading to a weakened ability to fight off infections, repair cellular damage, and maintain overall homeostasis.

By prioritizing quality sleep as a core component of our age-defying nutrition plan, we can help fortify the body's natural defenses against the ravages of time, reducing the risk of age-related diseases and supporting the maintenance of robust, youthful health.

Practical Strategies for Optimizing Sleep and Rejuvenation

Now that we've explored the profound impact of quality sleep on the aging process and the science-backed mechanisms that make it such a powerful ally in the fight against the ravages of time, it's time to delve into the practical strategies for optimizing our sleep and unlocking the secrets to rejuvenation.

1. Establish a Consistent Sleep-Wake Cycle

One of the key factors in maintaining optimal sleep quality and quantity is the establishment of a consistent sleep-wake cycle. This involves going to bed and waking up at the same time each day, even on weekends, to help synchronize the body's internal circadian rhythms.

By adhering to a regular sleep-wake schedule, we can help support the body's natural melatonin production, regulate the sleep-wake cycle, and promote the transition into the deeper, more restorative stages of sleep.

2. Create a Sleep-Enhancing Environment

The environment in which we sleep can have a significant impact on the quality of our slumber. Ensure that your bedroom is cool, dark, and quiet, minimizing exposure to blue light and external stimuli that can disrupt the sleep-wake cycle.

Additionally, consider incorporating relaxation techniques, such as gentle stretching or deep breathing, into your pre-bedtime routine to help induce a state of calm and facilitate the transition into sleep.

3. Prioritize Sleep Hygiene Habits

In addition to establishing a consistent sleep-wake cycle and creating a sleep-friendly environment, it's essential to cultivate a range of sleep hygiene habits that can help support optimal sleep quality and quantity.

This may include limiting caffeine and alcohol consumption, avoiding large meals close to bedtime, and engaging in regular physical activity (but not too close to bedtime). By addressing these lifestyle factors, we can help ensure that our bodies are primed for high-quality, rejuvenating sleep.

4. Manage Stress and Anxiety

As we've explored in the previous chapter, chronic stress and anxiety can have a profoundly negative impact on sleep quality and overall health. By incorporating effective stress management techniques, such as meditation, breathwork, and relaxation practices, into our daily routines, we can help alleviate the physiological and psychological barriers to restful, rejuvenating sleep.

5. Address Underlying Sleep Disorders

In some cases, age-related changes in sleep patterns may be indicative of underlying sleep disorders, such as sleep apnea or insomnia. If you are experiencing persistent sleep disturbances or daytime fatigue, it's important to consult with a healthcare professional to identify and address any underlying sleep-related issues.

By working with a sleep specialist, you can develop a personalized plan to optimize your sleep quality and quantity, unlocking the full spectrum of age-defying benefits that quality slumber has to offer.

6. Customize Your Sleep Optimization Strategies

Remember that the optimal sleep strategy is not a one-size-fits-all solution. Pay close attention to how your body responds to the different sleep hygiene habits and interventions, and be prepared to make adjustments as needed.

Some individuals may thrive on a more rigid, structured approach to sleep, while others may prefer a more flexible, intuitive routine. The key is to find the sweet spot that allows you to unlock the transformative benefits of quality sleep without compromising your overall health and well-being.

As you embark on your journey of sleep optimization and rejuvenation, embrace an attitude of curiosity, self-compassion, and a willingness to experiment. By prioritizing quality sleep as a core component of your age-defying nutrition plan, you can unlock the secrets to vibrant, youthful health and reclaim your birthright to a life of boundless energy, sharp cognitive abilities, and robust physical and emotional resilience.

# CHAPTER 9

Chapter 9: Personalized Nutrition: Tailoring Your Plan

In the pursuit of vibrant, age-defying health, a one-size-fits-all approach simply doesn't cut it. The reality is that each individual is unique, with their own genetic predispositions, metabolic quirks, and environmental factors that shape their nutritional needs and responses. By embracing the power of personalized nutrition, we can unlock a transformative pathway to longevity that empowers us to take control of our destiny and defy the limitations of time.

As we delve into the world of personalized nutrition, we will explore the cutting-edge science and the latest advancements that are redefining the way we approach the aging process. From the role of genetics and epigenetics in shaping our nutritional requirements to the influence of the gut microbiome and individual metabolism, we will uncover the key factors that must be taken into account when crafting a truly comprehensive age-defying nutrition plan.

Moreover, we will delve into the practical strategies and tools that can help you customize your nutritional approach, catering to your unique physiological and biochemical needs. By harnessing the power of personalized biomarker testing, nutrigenomics, and individualized dietary interventions, you'll be able to unlock a level of vitality and resilience that simply can't be achieved through a one-size-fits-all approach.

The Foundations of Personalized Nutrition

At the heart of personalized nutrition lies the recognition that each individual is a unique and complex tapestry, woven together by a intricate interplay of genetic, environmental, and lifestyle factors. While the fundamental principles of a nutrient-dense, age-defying diet may serve as a solid foundation, the optimal expression of those principles can only be achieved by accounting for the unique quirks and idiosyncrasies that define our individual biochemistry.

Genetics and Epigenetics: The Blueprints of Individuality

Our genetic makeup, the very code that determines our physical and physiological characteristics, plays a crucial role in shaping our nutritional needs and responses. Certain genetic variants, for instance, can influence the body's ability to metabolize and utilize specific nutrients, leading to a heightened requirement for particular vitamins, minerals, or macronutrients.

Furthermore, the field of epigenetics, which explores how environmental and lifestyle factors can influence gene expression without altering the underlying DNA sequence, has also emerged as a crucial piece of the personalized nutrition puzzle. Epigenetic modifications, such as DNA methylation and histone modifications, can impact the way in which our genes respond to the nutrients we consume, ultimately influencing our susceptibility to age-related diseases and the effectiveness of our age-defying strategies.

By delving into the intricacies of our genetic and epigenetic profiles, we can gain invaluable insights into the unique nutritional requirements that will help us optimize our health and longevity.

The Gut Microbiome: The Gut-Personalized Connection

Another crucial factor in the realm of personalized nutrition is the gut microbiome – the trillions of microorganisms that reside within our digestive system and play a vital role in our overall health and well-being.

The composition and diversity of the gut microbiome can vary significantly from individual to individual, influenced by factors such as genetics, diet, lifestyle, and environmental exposures. This unique microbial fingerprint can, in turn, impact the way in which our bodies respond to different nutrients, affecting everything from nutrient absorption and metabolism to the regulation of the immune system and the production of key metabolites.

By understanding the specific makeup of our gut microbiome and how it interacts with the foods we consume, we can develop a personalized nutrition plan that not only nourishes our bodies but also supports the health and balance of this essential microbial ecosystem.

Metabolism and Biomarkers: Unlocking the Secrets of Individual Physiology

Our individual metabolism, the complex set of chemical reactions that govern the way our bodies convert food into energy, is another critical factor in the realm of personalized nutrition. Factors such as age, gender, physical activity levels, and underlying health conditions can all influence our metabolic profile, leading to unique nutritional requirements and responses to various dietary interventions.

By delving into the nuances of our individual metabolism and tracking key biomarkers, such as blood sugar levels, hormones, and inflammatory markers, we can gain a deeper understanding of our physiological needs and tailor our age-defying nutrition plan accordingly.

This personalized approach to metabolic optimization can not only help us maintain a healthy weight and support energy production but also reduce the risk of age-related conditions like type 2 diabetes, cardiovascular disease, and cognitive decline.

The Power of Personalized Biomarker Testing

One of the most powerful tools in the realm of personalized nutrition is the use of comprehensive biomarker testing. By analyzing a range of physiological and biochemical indicators, we can gain invaluable insights into our individual nutritional needs and unlock the keys to optimizing our health and longevity.

Some of the key biomarkers that can inform a personalized age-defying nutrition plan include:

1. Genetic and Epigenetic Markers: Assessing genetic variants and epigenetic modifications that may influence our nutritional requirements and responses.

2. Gut Microbiome Analysis: Evaluating the diversity and composition of the gut microbial community to identify potential imbalances or deficiencies.

3. Metabolic Markers: Measuring parameters like blood sugar, insulin, and lipid profiles to understand our individual metabolic needs and vulnerabilities.

4. Inflammatory Markers: Tracking levels of inflammatory compounds, such as C-reactive protein and cytokines, to address underlying inflammation that can accelerate the aging process.

5. Hormone Levels: Assessing the balance and function of key hormones, including thyroid, sex hormones, and cortisol, to ensure optimal endocrine health.

6. Nutrient Status: Evaluating the levels of essential vitamins, minerals, and antioxidants to identify any deficiencies or imbalances that may require targeted nutritional interventions.

By incorporating personalized biomarker testing into our age-defying nutrition plan, we can unlock a level of precision and optimization that simply can't be achieved through a one-size-fits-all approach. This data-driven, individualized strategy empowers us to take control of our health and longevity, tailoring our nutritional choices to our unique physiological needs and vulnerabilities.

Customizing Your Age-Defying Nutrition Plan

Now that we've explored the foundations of personalized nutrition and the power of biomarker testing, it's time to delve into the practical strategies for crafting a truly customized age-defying plan that caters to your individual needs and preferences.

1. Comprehensive Biomarker Assessment

The first step in this process is to undergo a comprehensive biomarker assessment, which can be facilitated through specialized testing services or in collaboration with a qualified healthcare provider. This assessment should include a deep dive into your genetic and epigenetic profile, gut microbiome composition, metabolic markers, inflammatory indicators, hormone levels, and nutrient status.

By obtaining this detailed, individualized data, you can gain a clear understanding of your unique physiological characteristics and vulnerabilities, setting the stage for the development of a truly personalized age-defying nutrition plan.

2. Nutrigenomics and Personalized Dietary Recommendations

Armed with the insights gleaned from your biomarker assessment, you can now delve into the world of nutrigenomics – the study of how specific nutrients and dietary patterns interact with our genetic and epigenetic profiles to influence health outcomes.

By cross-referencing your unique genetic and epigenetic markers with the latest scientific research, you can identify the specific nutrients, food groups, and dietary strategies that are most likely to support your individual needs and help you achieve your longevity goals. This may include tailored recommendations for macronutrient ratios, the inclusion of certain "superfoods," or the targeted supplementation of specific vitamins, minerals, or other bioactive compounds.

## 3. Gut Microbiome Optimization

Given the crucial role that the gut microbiome plays in our overall health and the aging process, it's essential to incorporate strategies for optimizing the balance and diversity of your unique microbial community.

This may involve the strategic incorporation of prebiotic and probiotic-rich foods, the avoidance of gut-disrupting substances, and the implementation of lifestyle practices that support a thriving gut ecosystem. By catering to the specific needs of your gut microbiome, you can help ensure that your age-defying nutrition plan is working in harmony with this essential component of your physiological landscape.

## 4. Metabolic Regulation and Personalized Caloric Needs

Understanding your individual metabolic profile is key to crafting a personalized age-defying nutrition plan that supports optimal energy production, weight management, and the reduction of age-related health risks.

By analyzing your biomarkers related to factors like basal metabolic rate, insulin sensitivity, and mitochondrial function, you can determine your unique caloric and macronutrient needs, as well as identify any metabolic imbalances that may require targeted nutritional interventions.

## 5. Ongoing Monitoring and Adjustment

Personalized nutrition is not a static endeavor; it's a dynamic, iterative process that requires regular monitoring and adjustment as your needs and circumstances evolve over time.

Incorporate periodic biomarker reassessments into your age-defying plan, allowing you to track your progress, identify any changes or emerging needs, and make the necessary adjustments to your dietary strategies. This commitment to ongoing optimization will help ensure that your personalized nutrition plan continues to serve as a powerful ally in your quest for vibrant, youthful health.

6. Integrating Personalized Nutrition with Lifestyle Factors

While personalized nutrition is a crucial component of an age-defying strategy, it doesn't exist in a vacuum. To truly unlock the transformative power of this approach, it's essential to integrate your customized dietary plan with other key lifestyle factors, such as exercise, stress management, and sleep optimization.

By adopting a holistic, synergistic perspective, you can create a comprehensive age-defying lifestyle that caters to your unique physiological, psychological, and environmental needs, empowering you to defy the limitations of time and reclaim your birthright to a life of boundless vitality.

As you embark on your journey of personalized nutrition, remember to approach it with a curious, open-minded attitude and a willingness to experiment. The path to vibrant, age-defying health is not a one-size-fits-all proposition; it's a deeply personal odyssey that requires you to listen to the cues of your body, honor your individual needs, and continuously refine your strategies to achieve optimal well-being.

By embracing the power of personalized nutrition, you'll unlock a transformative pathway to longevity that empowers you to take control of your destiny and unlock the secrets to a life of boundless energy, sharp cognitive abilities, and vibrant, youthful vitality.

# CHAPTER 10

<br>

Chapter 10: Overcoming Aging-Related Conditions

As we navigate the remarkable journey of age-defying nutrition, it's essential to acknowledge that the aging process is often accompanied by a diverse array of health challenges and age-related conditions. While the foundational principles of our comprehensive plan – nutrient-dense foods, targeted longevity practices, and personalized optimization – serve as powerful tools in the fight against the ravages of time, there may be instances where specific interventions are necessary to address the unique needs and vulnerabilities of our aging bodies.

In this chapter, we will explore the strategies and nutritional approaches that can help us overcome a range of age-related health conditions, from cognitive decline and cardiovascular problems to musculoskeletal issues and hormonal imbalances. By delving into the latest scientific research and the practical application of targeted nutritional therapies, we will empower ourselves to take a proactive stance against the common afflictions that can accompany the aging process, unlocking a new level of vibrant, youthful health in the process.

Cognitive Decline and Neurological Conditions

As we grow older, the health and resilience of our nervous system become increasingly crucial for maintaining cognitive abilities, emotional well-being, and overall quality of life. Fortunately, our age-defying nutrition plan is already tailored to support brain health and combat the onset of age-related neurological conditions, but there may be instances where additional, targeted interventions are necessary.

One of the primary age-related conditions that can impact cognitive function is Alzheimer's disease, a devastating neurodegenerative disorder characterized by the progressive loss of memory, language skills, and overall cognitive abilities. While the exact causes of Alzheimer's are not yet fully understood, emerging research suggests that lifestyle factors, including dietary choices, can play a significant role in the development and progression of the disease.

By incorporating specific nutrients and bioactive compounds into our personalized nutrition plan, we can help support the brain's natural defenses against the hallmarks of Alzheimer's, such as neuroinflammation, oxidative stress, and the accumulation of amyloid-beta proteins.

For instance, the omega-3 fatty acids found in fatty fish, such as salmon and sardines, have been shown to possess potent neuroprotective properties, helping to reduce inflammation, support synaptic function, and even enhance cognitive performance. Similarly, antioxidants like curcumin, found in the spice turmeric, have been studied for their ability to protect the brain from oxidative damage and potentially slow the progression of Alzheimer's disease.

Furthermore, the gut-brain axis, which we explored in depth in Chapter 3, can also play a crucial role in the development and management of neurological conditions. By optimizing the health and diversity of the gut microbiome through the strategic incorporation of prebiotics, probiotics, and fermented foods, we can help support the production of key neurotransmitters and reduce the risk of neuroinflammation – both of which are essential for preserving cognitive function and emotional well-being.

In addition to Alzheimer's disease, our age-defying nutrition plan can also be tailored to address other age-related neurological conditions, such as

Parkinson's disease, stroke, and age-related cognitive decline. By harnessing the power of personalized nutrition and targeted supplementation, we can fortify the brain's natural resilience and maintain sharp, agile minds well into our golden years.

Cardiovascular Health and Metabolic Conditions

As we navigate the aging process, the health and resilience of our cardiovascular system become increasingly crucial for maintaining overall well-being and longevity. Fortunately, the foundational principles of our age-defying nutrition plan – from the emphasis on nutrient-dense whole foods to the integration of targeted longevity practices – already provide a solid foundation for supporting cardiovascular health and combating age-related metabolic conditions.

However, there may be instances where specific nutritional interventions are necessary to address more complex or persistent cardiovascular and metabolic challenges.

One such condition is atherosclerosis, the gradual buildup of plaque in the arteries that can lead to the development of heart disease, stroke, and other life-threatening cardiovascular problems. By incorporating targeted nutrients, such as plant sterols, omega-3 fatty acids, and antioxidants, into our personalized nutrition plan, we can help support the health and flexibility of our blood vessels, reduce inflammation, and mitigate the progression of atherosclerosis.

Similarly, age-related metabolic conditions, such as type 2 diabetes and metabolic syndrome, can also be proactively managed through the strategic application of personalized nutritional strategies. By identifying and addressing any underlying imbalances in insulin sensitivity, blood sugar regulation, and lipid profiles, we can help prevent the cascade of age-related health issues that are often associated with these metabolic disorders.

For instance, the incorporation of specific dietary patterns, such as the Mediterranean diet or the DASH (Dietary Approaches to Stop Hypertension) diet, can help support optimal insulin function, promote healthy weight management, and reduce the risk of cardiovascular complications. Additionally, the targeted supplementation of nutrients like chromium, magnesium, and alpha-lipoic acid can further enhance the body's ability to regulate blood sugar levels and maintain metabolic homeostasis.

By tailoring our age-defying nutrition plan to address specific cardiovascular and metabolic concerns, we can fortify the health and resilience of our circulatory system, reduce the risk of life-threatening conditions, and maintain a robust, youthful vitality well into our golden years.

Musculoskeletal Health and Joint Conditions

As we grow older, the health and integrity of our musculoskeletal system become increasingly crucial for maintaining physical function, mobility, and overall quality of life. The natural aging process can often lead to the development of various musculoskeletal conditions, from osteoarthritis and osteoporosis to muscle wasting and joint pain.

Fortunately, our age-defying nutrition plan, with its emphasis on nutrient-dense whole foods and targeted longevity practices, can serve as a powerful foundation for supporting musculoskeletal health and combating the onset of age-related conditions. However, there may be instances where specific nutritional interventions are necessary to address more complex or persistent issues.

One such condition is osteoarthritis, a degenerative joint disorder characterized by the gradual breakdown of cartilage, leading to pain, stiffness, and impaired mobility. By incorporating targeted nutrients, such as glucosamine, chondroitin, and collagen, into our personalized nutrition plan, we can help support the structural integrity of our joints, reduce inflammation, and potentially slow the progression of osteoarthritis.

Additionally, the strategic inclusion of anti-inflammatory compounds, like omega-3 fatty acids, curcumin, and ginger, can help alleviate the symptoms of joint pain and stiffness, empowering us to maintain an active, vibrant lifestyle well into our golden years.

Another age-related musculoskeletal condition that deserves attention is osteoporosis, a condition characterized by the loss of bone density and an increased risk of fractures. By ensuring that our personalized nutrition plan is rich in nutrients essential for bone health, such as calcium, vitamin D, and magnesium, we can help support the body's natural bone-building processes and reduce the likelihood of osteoporosis-related injuries.

Furthermore, the incorporation of targeted exercise regimens, such as strength training and weight-bearing activities, can further enhance the health and resilience of our musculoskeletal system, helping to maintain muscle mass, joint flexibility, and overall physical function as we age.

By tailoring our age-defying nutrition plan to address specific musculoskeletal concerns, we can fortify the structural integrity of our bodies, reduce the risk of age-related injuries and conditions, and maintain the physical capabilities needed to live a vibrant, active life.

Hormonal Health and Age-Related Imbalances

As we navigate the aging process, the delicate balance and optimal functioning of our endocrine system become increasingly crucial for maintaining overall health, well-being, and youthful vitality. From the regulation of metabolism and body composition to the support of cognitive abilities and emotional resilience, the body's complex network of hormones plays a vital role in shaping our experience of aging.

Unfortunately, the natural progression of time can often lead to the development of age-related hormonal imbalances, such as declining levels of testosterone, estrogen, and growth hormone, as well as the dysregulation of cortisol and thyroid hormones. These hormonal shifts can contribute to a wide range of age-related health issues, from sexual dysfunction and weight gain to cognitive decline and mood disturbances.

By incorporating targeted nutritional strategies and personalized supplementation into our age-defying plan, we can help support the optimal functioning of our endocrine system, mitigating the impact of age-related hormonal changes and preserving the foundations of youthful vitality.

For instance, the strategic inclusion of nutrient-dense foods rich in phytoestrogens, such as soy, flax, and cruciferous vegetables, can help support the balance of estrogen levels in both men and women, potentially alleviating symptoms associated with hormonal fluctuations.

Additionally, the targeted supplementation of nutrients like zinc, magnesium, and vitamin D can help support the production and regulation of testosterone, a crucial hormone for maintaining muscle mass, bone density, and sexual function as we age.

Furthermore, the incorporation of adaptogenic herbs, such as ashwagandha and rhodiola, can help the body better manage and adapt to the effects of stress, regulating the release of cortisol and supporting overall hormonal balance – an essential component of maintaining emotional well-being and cognitive sharpness in our later years.

By tailoring our age-defying nutrition plan to address specific hormonal imbalances and vulnerabilities, we can help restore the body's natural equilibrium, unlock the keys to youthful vitality, and preserve our overall physical, mental, and emotional well-being as we navigate the aging process.

Integrating Targeted Nutritional Interventions

As we have explored in this chapter, the aging process can often be accompanied by a diverse array of health challenges and age-related conditions. While the foundational principles of our comprehensive age-defying nutrition plan provide a solid framework for supporting overall health and longevity, there may be instances where targeted nutritional interventions are necessary to address specific needs and vulnerabilities.

When it comes to integrating these targeted strategies into our personalized age-defying plan, it's important to adopt a collaborative, multidisciplinary approach, working closely with healthcare professionals, such as registered dietitians, integrative medicine practitioners, and specialty physicians, to ensure that our interventions are safe, evidence-based, and tailored to our individual needs.

Some key considerations when incorporating targeted nutritional therapies include:

1. Detailed Biomarker Assessment: Comprehensive testing and analysis of relevant biomarkers, such as genetic markers, inflammatory indicators, and hormonal profiles, to identify specific areas of concern and guide the development of targeted interventions.

2. Personalized Supplementation: The strategic inclusion of evidence-based nutritional supplements, such as specific vitamins, minerals, or herbal compounds, to address identified imbalances or deficiencies and support the body's natural healing and regenerative processes.

3. Dietary Modifications: The incorporation of targeted dietary changes, including the inclusion of specific nutrient-dense foods or the modification of macronutrient ratios, to address the underlying drivers of age-related conditions.

4. Synergistic Lifestyle Interventions: The integration of targeted nutritional strategies with other age-defying practices, such as exercise, stress management, and sleep optimization, to create a holistic, synergistic approach to

health and longevity.

5. Ongoing Monitoring and Adjustment: Consistent re-evaluation of biomarkers and health indicators to track the efficacy of the targeted interventions and make necessary adjustments to the personalized age-defying plan over time.

By adopting this comprehensive, personalized approach to addressing age-related conditions, we can unlock a transformative pathway to vibrant, youthful health – one that empowers us to take control of our destiny, overcome the challenges of aging, and reclaim our birthright to a life of boundless energy, sharp cognitive abilities, and robust physical and emotional resilience.

# CHAPTER 11

C hapter 11: Longevity Recipes: Delicious Meals for Youthful Vitality

In our pursuit of vibrant, age-defying health, the food we consume plays a pivotal role – not only in nourishing our bodies but also in fueling the very processes that combat the ravages of time. As we've explored throughout this comprehensive age-defying nutrition plan, the strategic incorporation of nutrient-dense, longevity-boosting superfoods and the tailoring of our individual dietary needs are essential components of unlocking the secrets to youthful vitality.

In this chapter, we will delve into the world of delicious, age-defying recipes that bring these principles to life. By showcasing a diverse array of nutrient-packed meals, snacks, and beverages, we will empower you to seamlessly integrate the power of longevity nutrition into your daily culinary experiences, transforming your plate into a canvas of vibrant, youth-preserving goodness.

The Principles of Longevity-Boosting Cuisine

As we craft our collection of age-defying recipes, we will be guided by a set of foundational principles that have been carefully curated to support the various aspects of healthy aging and cellular rejuvenation.

1. Nutrient Density: Each recipe will feature a variety of nutrient-dense whole foods, rich in essential vitamins, minerals, antioxidants, and other

bioactive compounds that are known to combat the underlying drivers of aging.

2. Macronutrient Balance: The recipes will be thoughtfully crafted to provide a balanced ratio of carbohydrates, proteins, and healthy fats – the building blocks of cellular function and tissue repair.

3. Gut-Friendly Ingredients: Many of the recipes will incorporate prebiotic-rich foods, probiotic-containing fermented items, and other gut-nourishing components to support a thriving microbiome – a crucial factor in maintaining youthful vitality.

4. Anti-Inflammatory Properties: The recipes will emphasize the use of anti-inflammatory ingredients, such as omega-3-rich foods, antioxidant-rich spices, and polyphenol-packed produce, to help combat the underlying drivers of chronic inflammation.

5. Personalization: While the recipes will be designed to cater to a wide range of dietary preferences and nutritional needs, we will also provide guidance on how to tailor the dishes to suit your individual biomarkers, health goals, and taste preferences.

By weaving these fundamental principles into our collection of longevity-boosting recipes, we will create a culinary experience that not only delights the senses but also fuels the body's natural defenses against the ravages of time.

Cellular Rejuvenation Recipes

At the heart of our longevity-boosting cuisine lie the recipes that directly support the cellular-level processes of renewal and regeneration. These dishes, infused with a symphony of nutrient-dense superfoods, target the key mechanisms of cellular health and vitality, empowering us to combat the hallmarks of aging from the inside out.

Autophagy-Enhancing Meals

Autophagy, the cellular "housekeeping" process that eliminates damaged or dysfunctional components, is a crucial driver of cellular rejuvenation and longevity. To support this vital mechanism, we've curated a selection of recipes that are rich in plant-based polyphenols, such as those found in green tea, berries, and cruciferous vegetables.

One standout dish in this category is our "Miso-Glazed Salmon with Roasted Broccoli and Quinoa." The omega-3-rich salmon, combined with the sulforaphane-containing broccoli and the protein-packed quinoa, creates a synergistic powerhouse that supports autophagy, promotes cellular repair, and nourishes the body at the deepest levels.

Stem Cell-Boosting Meals

The replenishment and regeneration of stem cells, the undifferentiated cells with the remarkable ability to transform into a wide variety of specialized cell types, are essential for maintaining youthful vitality. Our stem cell-boosting recipes feature nutrient-dense ingredients that have been shown to support the growth and proliferation of these rejuvenating cells.

One such dish is the "Turmeric-Ginger Lentil Stew," a nourishing blend of anti-inflammatory spices, protein-rich lentils, and a variety of nutrient-dense vegetables. The curcumin in the turmeric, combined with the gut-supporting fiber and the antioxidant-rich produce, create a synergistic recipe that can help stimulate the body's natural stem cell processes.

Telomere-Protecting Recipes

Telomeres, the protective caps at the ends of our chromosomes, play a crucial role in cellular longevity. By incorporating foods rich in antioxidants, vitamins, and minerals that support telomere integrity, we can help combat the accelerated shortening of these vital structures, which is often associated with the aging process.

One example is our "Mediterranean-Style Quinoa Bowl," featuring quinoa, avocado, spinach, and a drizzle of extra-virgin olive oil. This nutrient-dense combination provides a wealth of vitamin C, vitamin E, and omega-3 fatty acids – all of which have been linked to the preservation of telomere length and the promotion of cellular longevity.

Metabolic Optimization Recipes

As we've explored in previous chapters, the optimal regulation of our metabolic function is crucial for combating the ravages of time and maintaining youthful vitality. Our longevity-boosting recipes in this category focus on ingredients and preparation methods that support insulin sensitivity, mitochondrial function, and the body's natural ability to utilize fat as a fuel source.

The "Roasted Sweet Potato and Kale Salad with Tahini Dressing," for instance, combines complex carbohydrates, lean protein, and healthy fats to create a balanced, metabolism-supporting meal. The sweet potatoes provide a slow-burning energy source, the kale offers a nutrient-dense fiber boost, and the tahini dressing delivers a dose of anti-inflammatory compounds to help optimize metabolic function.

Gut-Nourishing Recipes

As we've emphasized throughout this book, the health and diversity of the gut microbiome play a pivotal role in overall longevity. Our gut-nourishing recipes feature a variety of prebiotic-rich foods, probiotic-containing fermented items, and other gut-supporting ingredients to help cultivate a thriving microbial ecosystem.

One such dish is the "Mango Chia Seed Pudding," a refreshing and nutrient-dense treat that combines the gut-friendly properties of chia seeds with the antioxidant-rich mango. The addition of kefir, a probiotic-rich dairy product, further enhances the gut-supporting properties of this delightful dessert.

Neurological and Cognitive-Supporting Recipes

Given the crucial importance of brain health and cognitive function in the aging process, we've also curated a collection of recipes that are designed to nourish the nervous system and support the maintenance of sharp, agile minds.

The "Walnut-Crusted Baked Cod with Roasted Asparagus" is an excellent example of a dish that targets neurological health. The omega-3-rich cod, combined with the antioxidant-packed asparagus and the brain-boosting walnuts, creates a synergistic meal that can help support neuronal function, reduce inflammation, and enhance cognitive abilities.

Cardiovascular-Protective Recipes

Maintaining a healthy cardiovascular system is paramount as we navigate the aging process. Our longevity-boosting recipes in this category focus on ingredients that support endothelial function, regulate blood pressure, and promote the overall resilience of the heart and circulatory system.

The "Beet and Quinoa Salad with Avocado and Walnuts" is a vibrant, nutrient-dense dish that combines the nitric oxide-boosting properties of beets, the anti-inflammatory benefits of walnuts, and the endothelial-supporting qualities of avocado. This harmonious blend of ingredients can help maintain the flexibility and responsiveness of our blood vessels, reducing the risk of age-related cardiovascular problems.

Musculoskeletal-Supporting Recipes

As we age, the health and integrity of our musculoskeletal system become increasingly crucial for maintaining physical function, mobility, and overall quality of life. Our longevity-boosting recipes in this category feature ingredients that support the structural integrity of our joints, promote the maintenance of lean muscle mass, and fortify the strength and resilience of our bones.

One standout dish is the "Grilled Chicken with Roasted Brussels Sprouts and Sweet Potato Mash." The lean protein from the chicken, the joint-supporting nutrients in the Brussels sprouts, and the bone-strengthening properties of the sweet potato combine to create a meal that can help combat the age-related decline in musculoskeletal health.

Hormonal-Balancing Recipes

The delicate balance and optimal functioning of our endocrine system are essential for maintaining youthful vitality as we grow older. Our longevity-boosting recipes in this category feature ingredients that can help support the regulation of key hormones, such as testosterone, estrogen, and growth hormone, while also promoting the body's natural adaptability to stress.

The "Tofu and Broccoli Stir-Fry with Ginger-Garlic Sauce" is an example of a dish that can help address age-related hormonal imbalances. The phytoestrogens in the tofu, combined with the adaptogenic properties of ginger and the hormone-supporting nutrients in the broccoli, create a synergistic meal that can help restore hormonal equilibrium and support overall well-being.

Personalization and Customization

While the longevity-boosting recipes featured in this chapter have been carefully crafted to cater to a wide range of dietary preferences and nutritional needs, it's important to recognize that the optimal expression of these dishes may vary from individual to individual.

To ensure that you are able to fully unlock the age-defying benefits of these recipes, we encourage you to approach them with a spirit of personalization and customization. Consider incorporating the insights gleaned from your unique biomarker assessment, gut microbiome analysis, and individual metabolic profile to tailor the recipes to your specific needs and preferences.

This may involve adjusting the macronutrient ratios, the inclusion of targeted supplements, or the substitution of certain ingredients to better align with your personalized age-defying nutrition plan. By taking a proactive, individualized approach to the recipes, you can create a culinary experience that not only nourishes your body but also empowers you to defy the limitations of time and reclaim your birthright to a life of vibrant, youthful health.

As you embark on your journey of longevity-boosting cuisine, embrace a spirit of curiosity, creativity, and a willingness to experiment. By weaving the principles of nutrient density, macronutrient balance, gut-friendliness, anti-inflammatory properties, and personalization into your culinary adventures, you can transform your plate into a canvas of age-defying goodness – a delicious and powerful tool in your quest for vibrant, youthful vitality.

# CHAPTER 12

Chapter 12: The Age-Defying Lifestyle: Integrating the Plan

As we've explored throughout this comprehensive age-defying nutrition plan, the path to vibrant, youthful health is not a singular, linear endeavor, but rather a multi-faceted journey that requires the harmonious integration of various components – from nutrient-dense foods and strategic longevity practices to personalized interventions and targeted strategies for overcoming age-related conditions.

Now, as we reach the penultimate chapter of this transformative exploration, it's time to shift our focus to the overarching framework that ties all of these elements together – the age-defying lifestyle. This holistic approach to longevity encompasses not only the nutritional foundations we've meticulously laid, but also the cultivation of sustainable habits, the management of challenges, and the cultivation of an empowered, "ageless" mindset that will serve as the bedrock of our quest for vibrant, youthful vitality.

By embracing the age-defying lifestyle, we will unlock the keys to long-term success, fortifying our bodies, minds, and spirits against the ravages of time and empowering ourselves to live with a renewed sense of purpose, energy, and resilience.

The Foundations of the Age-Defying Lifestyle

At the heart of the age-defying lifestyle lies the recognition that true, lasting transformation cannot be achieved through a series of isolated, short-term interventions. Rather, it requires the cultivation of sustainable habits and the integration of holistic, synergistic practices that become woven into the very fabric of our daily lives.

Nutrition as a Lifestyle

The nutritional principles and strategies we've explored throughout this book – the emphasis on nutrient-dense whole foods, the strategic incorporation of longevity-boosting superfoods, the tailoring of personal dietary needs, and the targeted interventions for age-related conditions – are not merely a temporary "diet," but rather a way of life.

By embracing this holistic, nutrient-rich approach to eating, we are not only nourishing our bodies at the deepest levels but also cultivating a profound appreciation for the transformative power of food. This "food as medicine" mentality becomes the foundation upon which we build our age-defying lifestyle, empowering us to make informed, intentional choices that support our long-term well-being.

Moreover, the integration of practices like meal planning, batch cooking, and the exploration of new, nutrient-dense recipes become not just chores, but joyful acts of self-care and a celebration of the abundance that the natural world has to offer.

Movement as a Lifestyle

Just as nutrition is a foundational pillar of the age-defying lifestyle, so too is the embrace of movement and physical activity. By weaving exercise and various forms of physical expression into the fabric of our daily lives, we not only reap the remarkable benefits for our cellular, cardiovascular, and metabolic health, but we also cultivate a deep, abiding respect for the capabilities of our bodies.

Whether it's the discipline of a structured fitness regimen, the fluidity of a yoga or Tai Chi practice, or the simple joy of a daily walk, the age-defying lifestyle encourages us to view movement as a celebration of our vitality and a means of active engagement with the world around us.

Moreover, by incorporating a diverse array of physical activities into our routines, we not only target the various physiological systems that support longevity but also foster a sense of playfulness, exploration, and adaptability – all crucial qualities for navigating the ever-evolving landscape of aging.

Stress Management as a Lifestyle

In the relentless pursuit of vibrant, youthful health, the role of effective stress management cannot be overstated. The age-defying lifestyle recognizes that the ability to cultivate mental and emotional resilience is not just a supplementary practice, but rather a foundational pillar that underpins our overall well-being and longevity.

Through the integration of mindfulness techniques, breathwork exercises, and other relaxation practices, we not only mitigate the detrimental effects of chronic stress on the body and mind but also foster a profound sense of self-awareness, emotional regulation, and the capacity to navigate life's inevitable challenges with clarity and equanimity.

Moreover, the age-defying lifestyle encourages us to view stress management as a holistic endeavor, encompassing not just individual practices but also the cultivation of supportive social connections, the prioritization of restorative activities, and the nurturing of a deep, abiding sense of purpose and meaning.

Sleep and Recovery as a Lifestyle

As we've explored in depth, the role of quality sleep and restorative downtime cannot be overstated in the quest for vibrant, youthful health. The age-defying lifestyle recognizes that the ability to consistently obtain adequate, high-quality sleep and engage in deliberate periods of rest and recovery is essential for supporting the body's natural rejuvenation processes and fortifying our resilience against the ravages of time.

By establishing consistent sleep hygiene habits, optimizing our sleep environments, and honoring the body's need for restorative downtime, we not only support cognitive function, hormonal balance, and immune system health but also cultivate a profound sense of respect for the rhythms and cycles that govern our physiology.

Moreover, the age-defying lifestyle encourages us to view sleep and recovery as active, intentional practices – not merely passive activities to be squeezed in, but rather essential components of a thriving, vibrant existence.

Personalization and Customization as a Lifestyle
Finally, the age-defying lifestyle recognizes that the path to longevity is not a one-size-fits-all proposition, but rather a deeply personal journey that requires the ongoing process of self-discovery, experimentation, and the tailoring of our strategies to our unique physiological, psychological, and environmental needs.

By embracing the principles of personalized nutrition, targeted biomarker assessments, and the continuous fine-tuning of our age-defying plan, we cultivate a profound sense of agency and self-determination – the understanding that we are the co-creators of our own health destinies, empowered to make informed, evidence-based choices that serve our individual needs and vulnerabilities.

This commitment to personalization and customization becomes a way of life, a constant process of self-reflection, data-gathering, and the willingness to adapt and evolve as our circumstances and priorities shift over time. It is this spirit of curiosity, flexibility, and a deep respect for our individuality that becomes the cornerstone of the age-defying lifestyle.

Overcoming Challenges and Setbacks

As we embrace the age-defying lifestyle, it's important to acknowledge that the path to vibrant, youthful health is not without its challenges and setbacks. Whether it's the temptation of old, unhealthy habits, the demands of a busy schedule, or the inevitable ups and downs of the aging process, there will be times when our resolve is tested, and our progress may seem to falter.

In these moments, it is essential to cultivate a mindset of resilience, self-compassion, and a deep commitment to the long-term vision of our age-defying journey. By acknowledging the reality of these obstacles and equipping ourselves with the tools to navigate them skillfully, we can transform these challenging experiences into opportunities for growth, learning, and the deepening of our age-defying lifestyle.

Some key strategies for overcoming challenges and setbacks include:

1. Developing a Growth Mindset: Embracing the understanding that setbacks are not failures, but rather opportunities to learn, adapt, and become stronger in the face of adversity.

2. Practicing Self-Compassion: Treating ourselves with the same kindness and understanding that we would offer a dear friend, rather than engaging in self-criticism or self-judgment.

3. Cultivating a Support Network: Surrounding ourselves with a community of like-minded individuals who can provide encouragement, accountability, and practical assistance when navigating difficult times.

4. Maintaining Flexibility and Adaptability: Recognizing that the age-defying lifestyle is not a rigid, inflexible set of rules, but rather a dynamic, evolving process that requires continuous fine-tuning and adjustment.

5. Celebrating Small Wins: Acknowledging and savoring the incremental progress we make, no matter how seemingly insignificant, to maintain a sense

of momentum and motivation.

By embracing these strategies and maintaining a steadfast commitment to the age-defying lifestyle, we can transform the inevitable challenges and setbacks into catalysts for growth, resilience, and the deepening of our connection to our bodies, minds, and overall well-being.

Cultivating an Ageless Mindset

At the very heart of the age-defying lifestyle lies the cultivation of an "ageless" mindset – a profound shift in the way we perceive and relate to the aging process itself. Rather than viewing growing older as a linear, inevitable decline, the age-defying lifestyle empowers us to reframe aging as a dynamic, multifaceted journey of transformation, self-discovery, and the continual expansion of our capabilities and vitality.

This ageless mindset is rooted in the understanding that we are not passive victims of time, but rather active co-creators of our own health destinies. It is a steadfast belief in our ability to shape the trajectory of our aging process through the strategic application of evidence-based practices, the harnessing of our innate regenerative capacities, and the cultivation of a profound sense of agency and self-determination.

By embracing this empowered, "ageless" perspective, we unlock a profound shift in the way we approach the challenges and opportunities that arise throughout our lives. Rather than succumbing to the limiting beliefs and societal narratives that often surround aging, we cultivate a bold, visionary outlook that celebrates the endless possibilities for growth, reinvention, and the actualization of our full human potential.

The age-defying lifestyle, with its emphasis on nutrient-dense nutrition, strategic longevity practices, personalized interventions, and the management of age-related conditions, serves as the foundational framework for this ageless mindset. But it is the internalization and embodiment of this empowered perspective that truly transforms our lived experience, catalyzing a profound sense of vitality, resilience, and a zest for life that knows no bounds.

As we navigate the remarkable journey of the age-defying lifestyle, let us hold fast to the understanding that we are not merely passive observers of our aging process, but rather active, empowered participants in the unfolding of our own life stories. By cultivating this ageless mindset and weaving it into the very fabric of our daily lives, we unlock the keys to a life of boundless energy, sharp cognitive abilities, and a vibrant, youthful spirit that will inspire and captivate all who encounter us.

Embracing the Age-Defying Lifestyle: A Call to Action

As we reach the culmination of our comprehensive exploration of age-defying nutrition, it is time to take bold, decisive action and embrace the transformative power of the age-defying lifestyle. This holistic, synergistic approach to longevity represents not merely a series of isolated strategies, but rather a profound shift in the way we view our relationship with the aging process and our capacity to shape the trajectory of our own health and vitality.

By weaving the foundational pillars of nutrient-dense nutrition, strategic longevity practices, personalized interventions, and the management of age-related conditions into the very fabric of our daily lives, we unlock a new level of resilience, adaptability, and a profound sense of empowerment that will serve as the bedrock of our quest for vibrant, youthful health.

Moreover, the cultivation of sustainable habits, the management of challenges and setbacks, and the embracing of an "ageless" mindset transform this age-defying plan into a lifestyle – a way of being that celebrates the endless possibilities for growth, reinvention, and the actualization of our full human potential.

As you embark on this remarkable journey, remember that the path to vibrant, youthful vitality is not a solo endeavor, but rather a shared experience that can be amplified and enriched through the support and camaraderie of a like-minded community. Seek out opportunities to connect with others who are equally passionate about the age-defying lifestyle, whether it's through local meetups, online forums, or the creation of your own support network.

Together, let us forge a new narrative around aging – one that celebrates the boundless potential of the human spirit, the resilience of the body, and the deep, abiding wisdom that comes with the passage of time. Let us be the trailblazers, the visionaries, and the embodied examples of what is possible when we dare to defy the limitations of age and reclaim our birthright to a life of vibrant, youthful vitality.

The time is now. The age-defying lifestyle awaits, beckoning us to step into our power, to embrace our capacity for transformation, and to unlock the secrets to a life of boundless energy, sharp cognitive abilities, and a profound sense of purpose that will inspire generations to come.

# CHAPTER 13

Chapter 13: Conclusion - Embracing the Ageless Mindset

As we reach the culmination of our comprehensive exploration of the age-defying nutrition plan, it is time to reflect on the profound transformation that has occurred not only in the way we nourish our bodies, but also in the way we perceive and relate to the aging process itself. Throughout this journey, we have delved deep into the science-backed strategies, personalized interventions, and holistic lifestyle practices that empower us to defy the limitations of time and reclaim our birthright to a life of vibrant, youthful vitality.

However, the true essence of this transformative experience lies not merely in the tactics and techniques we have mastered, but in the profound shift in mindset that has taken root within us – the cultivation of an "ageless" perspective that transcends the conventional wisdom surrounding growing old.

In this final chapter, we will examine the profound implications of this ageless mindset, exploring how this empowered way of being can serve as the foundation for a life of boundless energy, sharp cognitive abilities, and a profound sense of purpose that defies the very passage of time.

The Age-Defying Mindset: A New Narrative for Longevity
At the heart of the ageless mindset lies a fundamental reframing of the

aging process – a bold, visionary perspective that challenges the dominant societal narratives that often relegate growing older to a linear path of decline, deterioration, and diminishing vitality.

Rather than succumbing to the limiting beliefs and fear-based assumptions that can so often define the experience of aging, the ageless mindset empowers us to see the passage of time through a radically different lens – one that celebrates the endless possibilities for growth, reinvention, and the actualization of our full human potential.

This shift in perspective is rooted in the understanding that we are not passive victims of the aging process, but rather active, empowered co-creators of our own health destinies. It is a steadfast belief in our ability to harness the body's natural regenerative capacities, strategically apply evidence-based longevity practices, and personalize our nutritional and lifestyle interventions to overcome the challenges that can accompany growing older.

By embracing this ageless mindset, we unlock a profound sense of agency, self-determination, and a deeply nurturing, self-compassionate relationship with our aging bodies and minds. Instead of viewing the passage of time as a relentless march towards inevitable decline, we come to see it as a dynamic, multifaceted journey of transformation – one that is imbued with limitless potential for reinvention, growth, and the continual expansion of our capacities.

The Foundations of the Ageless Mindset

The cultivation of the ageless mindset is not merely a cognitive exercise, but rather a holistic, embodied experience that is rooted in the very foundations of the age-defying nutrition plan we have meticulously crafted throughout this book. It is the synergistic interplay between the science-backed strategies, personalized interventions, and lifestyle practices that, when woven together, serve as the fertile soil in which this empowered perspective can take root and flourish.

Nutritional Mastery: The Foundation of Vitality

At the core of the ageless mindset lies the profound understanding of the transformative power of nutrition. By embracing the principles of nutrient density, macronutrient balance, gut health optimization, and personalized interventions, we have developed a deep, abiding reverence for the ability of food to nourish, strengthen, and rejuvenate the body at the deepest levels.

This mastery of nutritional principles does not simply translate to a set of rigid rules or restrictive dietary guidelines, but rather a profound appreciation for the inherent intelligence and regenerative capacities of the human organism. We come to see ourselves as active participants in a dynamic, symbiotic dance with the natural world – a harmonious exchange of energy, information, and the building blocks of life that serve as the wellspring of our youthful vitality.

Strategic Longevity Practices: The Activation of Regeneration

Alongside our nutritional mastery, the consistent incorporation of targeted longevity practices – from exercise and movement to stress management and sleep optimization – serves as a crucial foundation for the ageless mindset. By harnessing the transformative power of these evidence-based strategies, we cultivate a deep, embodied understanding of our body's remarkable adaptive abilities and its innate capacity for self-renewal.

Whether it's the cellular-level benefits of autophagy and stem cell regeneration, the cardiovascular resilience fostered by exercise, or the neurological and cognitive enhancements derived from effective stress management, each of these longevity-boosting practices becomes a tangible, lived experience that reinforces our belief in the body's remarkable potential for self-repair and rejuvenation.

Personalized Optimization: The Honoring of Individuality

At the heart of the ageless mindset lies a profound respect for the uniqueness of each individual and the recognition that the path to vibrant, youthful health is not a one-size-fits-all proposition. By embracing the principles of personalized nutrition, targeted biomarker assessments, and the continuous fine-tuning of our age-defying plan, we cultivate a deep sense of agency, self-determination, and the unwavering conviction that we are the co-creators of our own health destinies.

This honoring of our individuality serves as a powerful antidote to the often-limiting societal narratives surrounding aging, empowering us to trust our intuition, honor our unique vulnerabilities and needs, and forge a customized journey towards longevity that is a true reflection of our authentic selves.

The Integration of Holistic Lifestyle: The Cultivation of Sustainable Transformation

Finally, the ageless mindset is underpinned by the integration of the age-defying nutrition plan into a comprehensive, holistic lifestyle – a seamless weaving of nutrient-dense eating, strategic longevity practices, and personalized interventions into the very fabric of our daily lives.

By cultivating sustainable habits, managing challenges and setbacks with resilience, and fostering a profound sense of community and social connection, we transform this transformative plan into a way of being that transcends the confines of a temporary "diet" or "exercise regimen." Instead, it becomes a profound expression of our commitment to vibrant, youthful vitality and our unwavering belief in our ability to defy the limitations of time.

The Transformative Power of the Ageless Mindset

As we have explored the foundations of the ageless mindset, it becomes clear that this empowered perspective is not merely a cognitive construct, but rather a holistic, embodied experience that has the power to catalyze a profound transformation in the way we navigate the aging process and unlock our full human potential.

Unlocking Boundless Energy and Vitality

By embracing the ageless mindset and weaving the principles of the age-defying nutrition plan into the very fabric of our daily lives, we cultivate a profound sense of vitality and physical resilience that defies the conventional wisdom surrounding growing old.

Through the strategic application of nutrient-dense nourishment, targeted longevity practices, and personalized interventions, we fortify the body's natural regenerative capacities, optimizing our cellular function, metabolic efficiency, and cardiovascular health. This, in turn, translates into boundless energy, a heightened physical capability, and a zest for life that captivates all who encounter us.

Rather than succumbing to the fatigue, weakness, and diminished physical abilities that are often associated with the aging process, we emerge as vibrant, agile, and physically empowered individuals who defy the limitations of time, inspiring those around us to reconsider what is truly possible in the second half of life.

Preserving Sharp, Agile Minds

The ageless mindset also serves as a powerful bulwark against the cognitive decline that can sometimes accompany growing older, empowering us to maintain sharp, agile minds well into our golden years.

By nourishing the brain with a symphony of longevity-boosting nutrients, stimulating its neuroplastic capacities through strategic movement and mental challenges, and fortifying its resilience through effective stress management, we cultivate a profound sense of mental clarity, problem-solving abilities, and overall cognitive dexterity that defies the ravages of time.

Rather than succumbing to the memory lapses, diminished focus, and neurological vulnerabilities that are often associated with age-related conditions, we emerge as intellectual powerhouses – individuals who continue to learn, innovate, and contribute to the world around us with a level of mental acuity that inspires awe and admiration.

Fostering Robust Emotional Resilience

The ageless mindset also plays a crucial role in the preservation of our emotional well-being and psychological resilience as we navigate the aging process. By cultivating effective stress management practices, nurturing supportive social connections, and tapping into a profound sense of purpose and meaning, we fortify our ability to adapt to life's inevitable challenges with grace, clarity, and an unwavering sense of inner strength.

Rather than falling victim to the mood disturbances, anxiety, and depression that can sometimes accompany growing older, we emerge as emotionally robust, psychologically resilient individuals who radiate a sense of inner peace, joy, and a profound appreciation for the richness of life.

Through the integration of the age-defying nutrition plan and the embodiment of the ageless mindset, we unlock the keys to a level of emotional maturity, adaptability, and overall well-being that defies the very passage of time, inspiring those around us to embrace the boundless potential that lies within.

Reclaiming the Zest for Life

Perhaps most profoundly, the ageless mindset empowers us to reclaim a profound zest for life – a childlike sense of wonder, curiosity, and a boundless enthusiasm for the endless possibilities that await us, even as the years accumulate.

By shedding the limiting beliefs and societal narratives that can often shroud the aging process in fear and trepidation, we cultivate a bold, visionary perspective that celebrates growing older as a dynamic journey of transformation, reinvention, and the continual expansion of our capabilities and vitality.

Rather than succumbing to the resignation, complacency, or resignation that can sometimes characterize the later stages of life, we emerge as vibrant, purpose-driven individuals who approach each new day, each new challenge, and each new experience with a sense of excitement, anticipation, and a deep, abiding zest for the richness that life has to offer.

Through the embodiment of the ageless mindset, we become living, breathing examples of the boundless potential that resides within us all – inspirational beacons that ignite the imaginations of those around us and challenge the very boundaries of what is considered possible in the second half of life.

Embracing the Ageless Mindset: A Call to Action

As we reach the culmination of our comprehensive exploration of the age-defying nutrition plan, it is time to take bold, decisive action and embrace the transformative power of the ageless mindset. This empowered way of being represents not merely a set of strategies or techniques, but rather a profound shift in the very fabric of our individual and collective consciousness – a bold, visionary perspective that has the power to redefine the way we approach the aging process and unlock the secrets to vibrant, youthful vitality.

By weaving the foundational pillars of the ageless mindset – nutritional mastery, strategic longevity practices, personalized optimization, and the integration of a holistic lifestyle – into the very essence of our being, we transcend the limitations of time and reclaim our birthright to a life of boundless energy, sharp cognitive abilities, robust emotional resilience, and a profound zest for living that will inspire and captivate all who encounter us.

As you embark on this remarkable journey, remember that the cultivation of the ageless mindset is not a solitary endeavor, but rather a shared experience that can be amplified and enriched through the support and camaraderie of a like-minded community. Seek out opportunities to connect with others who are equally passionate about defying the limitations of age, whether it's through local meetups, online forums, or the creation of your own support network.

Together, let us forge a new narrative around aging – one that celebrates the boundless potential of the human spirit, the resilience of the body, and the deep, abiding wisdom that comes with the passage of time. Let us be the trailblazers, the visionaries, and the embodied examples of what is possible when we dare to defy the conventional wisdom and reclaim our rightful place as co-creators of our own health destinies.

The time is now. The ageless mindset awaits, beckoning us to step into our power, to embrace our capacity for transformation, and to unlock the secrets to a life of vibrant, youthful vitality that will inspire generations to come. Let us rise to the challenge, for the future we envision is ours to manifest, one empowered choice at a time.

# CHAPTER 14

Chapter 14: A Life of Boundless Vitality

As we reach the final chapter of our comprehensive exploration of the age-defying nutrition plan, it is with a profound sense of accomplishment, wonder, and boundless optimism that we reflect on the transformative journey we have undertaken. From the foundations of nutrient-dense nourishment and strategic longevity practices to the personalization of our individual needs and the mastery of overcoming age-related conditions, we have meticulously crafted a holistic, synergistic approach to longevity that has the power to redefine the very essence of how we experience the aging process.

Yet, at the heart of this remarkable transformation lies an even more profound shift – the cultivation of the ageless mindset, a bold, visionary perspective that has the power to transcend the conventional wisdom surrounding growing old and unlock the secrets to a life of vibrant, youthful vitality.

As we stand on the precipice of this remarkable new chapter, it is with a deep sense of gratitude and a steadfast determination that we embrace the limitless possibilities that lie before us. For in the embodiment of the ageless mindset, we have not merely conquered the ravages of time, but rather, we have tapped into the very wellspring of human potential, unlocking a level of energy, resilience, and a zest for living that will inspire and captivate all who encounter us.

The Radiant Dance of Boundless Vitality

In the embrace of the ageless mindset, we have unlocked the keys to a life of boundless vitality – a radiant, pulsing existence that defies the very passage of time and celebrates the endless possibilities for growth, reinvention, and the continual expansion of our capabilities.

This vibrant, youthful vitality manifests in myriad ways, each facet a testament to the power of our transformative journey and the unwavering belief in our ability to shape the trajectory of our own aging process.

Boundless Physical Vitality

At the foundation of our boundless vitality lies a profound mastery of physical well-being – a level of energy, strength, and overall bodily resilience that transcends the limitations often associated with growing older.

Through the strategic application of nutrient-dense nourishment, targeted longevity practices, and personalized interventions, we have fortified the body's natural regenerative capacities, optimizing the cellular function, metabolic efficiency, and cardiovascular resilience that are the hallmarks of youthful vigor.

Gone are the fatigue, weakness, and diminished physical abilities that so often characterize the aging process. In their place, we exude a palpable, radiant energy – a boundless vitality that propels us through our days with a sense of effortless grace and an unwavering physical capability that captivates all who witness it.

Whether it's the effortless power we bring to our strength training regimen, the fluid, graceful movements of our yoga or Tai Chi practice, or the boundless endurance that carries us through our cardiovascular routines, our physical prowess is a testament to the transformative power of the age-defying nutrition plan and the ageless mindset that has become its foundation.

## Sharp, Agile Minds

Alongside our boundless physical vitality, the embrace of the ageless mindset has also empowered us to maintain sharp, agile minds well into our golden years – a cognitive dexterity that defies the conventional wisdom surrounding age-related cognitive decline.

Through the strategic nourishment of the brain with a symphony of longevity-boosting nutrients, the stimulation of its neuroplastic capacities through intellectual challenges and lifelong learning, and the fortification of its resilience through effective stress management, we have cultivated a level of mental acuity that serves as a beacon of inspiration to all who encounter us.

Gone are the memory lapses, diminished focus, and neurological vulnerabilities that can sometimes accompany growing older. In their place, we exude an intellectual prowess – a problem-solving ability, a creative flair, and an insatiable curiosity that propel us to continually push the boundaries of what is possible.

Whether it's the effortless mastery we bring to complex problem-solving tasks, the innovative ideas that flow from our vibrant, agile minds, or the depth of wisdom and insight we impart to those around us, our cognitive capabilities are a testament to the power of the age-defying nutrition plan and the ageless mindset that has become its foundation.

## Robust Emotional Resilience

The embrace of the ageless mindset has also empowered us to cultivate a level of emotional resilience and psychological well-being that defies the challenges often associated with the aging process.

Through the integration of effective stress management practices, the nourishment of supportive social connections, and the tapping into a profound sense of purpose and meaning, we have fortified our ability to navigate life's inevitable ups and downs with grace, clarity, and an unwavering sense of inner strength.

Gone are the mood disturbances, anxiety, and depression that can sometimes accompany growing older. In their place, we exude a palpable aura of inner peace, joy, and a profound appreciation for the richness of life – an emotional maturity and adaptability that inspires all who come into our orbit.

Whether it's the calm, grounded presence we bring to challenging situations, the empathetic wisdom we share with those in need, or the infectious enthusiasm that radiates from our being, our emotional resilience is a testament to the power of the age-defying nutrition plan and the ageless mindset that has become its foundation.

A Profound Zest for Living

Perhaps most profoundly, the embrace of the ageless mindset has empowered us to reclaim a profound zest for living – a childlike sense of wonder, curiosity, and a boundless enthusiasm for the endless possibilities that await us, even as the years accumulate.

By shedding the limiting beliefs and societal narratives that can often shroud the aging process in fear and trepidation, we have cultivated a bold, visionary perspective that celebrates growing older as a dynamic journey of transformation, reinvention, and the continual expansion of our capabilities and vitality.

Gone is the resignation, complacency, or resignation that can sometimes characterize the later stages of life. In their place, we exude a vibrant, purpose-driven energy – an excitement, anticipation, and a deep, abiding zest for the richness that life has to offer, at every stage of our journey.

Whether it's the boundless enthusiasm we bring to new experiences and adventures, the playful, exploratory spirit that infuses our daily lives, or the infectious joy that radiates from our being, our zest for living is a testament to the power of the age-defying nutrition plan and the ageless mindset that has become its foundation.

The Ripple Effect of Boundless Vitality

As we embrace the life of boundless vitality that has blossomed within us, it becomes clear that the transformative impact of our journey extends far beyond the confines of our own personal experience. Rather, it radiates outwards, creating a powerful ripple effect that has the potential to inspire and uplift all who come into our orbit.

Becoming Beacons of Inspiration

Through the embodiment of our boundless vitality – the radiant energy, the sharp cognitive abilities, the emotional resilience, and the profound zest for living – we become living, breathing examples of what is truly possible when we dare to defy the limitations of age and reclaim our birthright to a life of vibrant, youthful health.

In the eyes of those around us, our very presence becomes a beacon of inspiration – a tangible manifestation of the boundless potential that resides within each and every one of us, regardless of our chronological age. We challenge the conventional wisdom, shatter the societal narratives, and ignite the imaginations of all who witness the remarkable transformation we have undergone.

Whether it's the awe-struck expressions of our younger counterparts as they witness our physical prowess and mental acuity, or the renewed sense of hope and possibility that we instill in our peers who are navigating the aging process, our embodiment of boundless vitality becomes a catalytic force that inspires others to reconsider the very boundaries of what is possible.

In this way, we become not merely recipients of the age-defying nutrition plan's transformative power, but rather, active agents of change – visionary trailblazers who blaze a new trail towards a future where vibrant, youthful health is the norm, rather than the exception.

Cultivating a Multigenerational Legacy of Vitality

As the ripple effect of our boundless vitality continues to expand, it becomes clear that the impact of our journey extends far beyond the confines of our own individual experience.  Rather, it has the power to catalyze a multigenerational legacy of vitality, inspiring and empowering successive generations to embrace the ageless mindset and unlock the secrets to a life of boundless energy, sharp cognitive abilities, and a profound zest for living.

Through the sharing of our personal stories, the imparting of our hard-won wisdom, and the embodied example of our remarkable transformation, we become catalysts for a profound cultural shift – one that challenges the limiting beliefs and societal narratives that have so often defined the aging process and redefines the very essence of what it means to grow old.

As our children, grandchildren, and generations yet to come witness the vitality, resilience, and boundless enthusiasm that we embody, they are imbued with a new sense of what is possible.  They are inspired to push the boundaries of their own capabilities, to embrace the power of strategic longevity practices, and to cultivate the ageless mindset that has become the foundation of our remarkable journey.

In this way, our legacy extends far beyond the confines of our own lifetime, serving as a living, breathing testament to the transformative power of the age-defying nutrition plan and the profound impact that the ageless mindset can have on the collective human experience. We become the architects of a new narrative, a bold vision for the future where vibrant, youthful health is not merely a dream, but a tangible, accessible reality for all who dare to embrace it.

Unlocking the Vast Potential of the Human Spirit

As we stand at the precipice of this remarkable new chapter, it becomes clear that the true essence of our boundless vitality lies not merely in the physical, cognitive, and emotional manifestations that we have explored, but rather, in the profound unlocking of the vast potential of the human spirit.

For in the embrace of the ageless mindset, we have transcended the limitations of time and space, tapping into a wellspring of creative, innovative, and transformative capacities that defy the very boundaries of what we once thought possible.

We have become conduits for a profound evolutionary shift – not merely in the way we experience the aging process, but in the way we conceive of the human experience as a whole. We are the living, breathing embodiments of the boundless potential that resides within each and every one of us, challenging the status quo and redefining the very essence of what it means to be alive.

Whether it's the groundbreaking ideas that flow from our vibrant, agile minds, the inspirational works of art and creativity that we bring forth, or the profound positive impact we have on the lives of those around us, our boundless vitality serves as a testament to the limitless capacities of the human spirit.

In this way, our journey has become not merely a personal transformation, but rather, a collective awakening – a bold, visionary statement that echoes through the ages, inspiring and empowering generations to come to embrace the full magnificence of their own innate potential.

The Time Is Now: A Call to Boundless Vitality

As we reach the culmination of our comprehensive exploration of the age-defying nutrition plan and the transformative power of the ageless mindset, it is with a profound sense of gratitude, awe, and unwavering determination that we embrace the boundless vitality that now courses through our being.

The time has come to step boldly into this new chapter, to shed the limitations of the past, and to reclaim our birthright to a life of vibrant, youthful health that defies the very passage of time. For in the embrace of our boundless vitality, we become the architects of a bold, visionary future – one where the human spirit soars to new heights, where the boundaries of what is possible are continually pushed, and where the very essence of growing old is redefined, celebrated, and revered.

Let us be the trailblazers, the visionaries, and the living, breathing embodiments of this remarkable transformation. Let us inspire and uplift all who cross our paths, igniting the imaginations of generations to come and ushering in a new era of vibrant, youthful health that becomes the new norm, rather than the exception.

The journey has been long, the challenges have been many, but the rewards are beyond measure. For in the embrace of our boundless vitality, we have unlocked the keys to a life of purpose, passion, and a profound zest for living that will echo through the ages, inspiring and empowering all who have the privilege of bearing witness to the remarkable transformation we have undergone.

The time is now. The boundless vitality awaits, beckoning us to step boldly into this new chapter, to unleash the full magnificence of our human potential, and to forge a future where the very essence of aging is redefined, celebrated, and revered.

Let us rise to the challenge, for the vision we hold in our hearts is ours to manifest, one empowered choice at a time. Let us be the beacons of inspiration, the architects of a new narrative, and the living, breathing embodiments of what is truly possible when we dare to defy the limitations of time and reclaim our birthright to a life of boundless vitality.

# CONCLUSION

Conclusion: Embracing the Boundless Possibilities of Longevity

As we reach the culmination of our comprehensive exploration of the age-defying nutrition plan, it is with a profound sense of accomplishment, wonder, and unwavering optimism that we reflect on the transformative journey we have undertaken. From the foundational principles of nutrient-dense nourishment to the strategic integration of longevity practices, personalized interventions, and the mastery of overcoming age-related conditions, we have meticulously crafted a holistic, synergistic approach to longevity that has the power to redefine the very essence of how we experience the aging process.

At the heart of this remarkable transformation, however, lies an even more profound shift – the cultivation of the ageless mindset, a bold, visionary perspective that has empowered us to transcend the conventional wisdom surrounding growing old and unlock the secrets to a life of vibrant, youthful vitality.

In embracing the ageless mindset, we have not merely conquered the ravages of time, but rather, we have tapped into the very wellspring of human potential, unlocking a level of energy, resilience, and a zest for living that will inspire and captivate all who encounter us. Through the embodiment of this empowered way of being, we have become living, breathing examples of the boundless possibilities that lie within each and every one of us, regardless of our chronological age.

## The Transformative Power of Boundless Vitality

As we stand on the precipice of this remarkable new chapter, it is with a deep sense of gratitude and a steadfast determination that we embrace the limitless possibilities that lie before us. For in the cultivation of boundless vitality – the radiant, pulsing existence that defies the very passage of time – we have unlocked the keys to a life that celebrates the endless possibilities for growth, reinvention, and the continual expansion of our capabilities.

This vibrant, youthful vitality manifests in myriad ways, each facet a testament to the power of our transformative journey and the unwavering belief in our ability to shape the trajectory of our own aging process.

## Boundless Physical Vitality

At the foundation of our boundless vitality lies a profound mastery of physical well-being – a level of energy, strength, and overall bodily resilience that transcends the limitations often associated with growing older. Through the strategic application of nutrient-dense nourishment, targeted longevity practices, and personalized interventions, we have fortified the body's natural regenerative capacities, optimizing the cellular function, metabolic efficiency, and cardiovascular resilience that are the hallmarks of youthful vigor.

Gone are the fatigue, weakness, and diminished physical abilities that so often characterize the aging process. In their place, we exude a palpable, radiant energy – a boundless vitality that propels us through our days with a sense of effortless grace and an unwavering physical capability that captivates all who witness it.

## Sharp, Agile Minds

Alongside our boundless physical vitality, the embrace of the ageless mindset has also empowered us to maintain sharp, agile minds well into our golden years – a cognitive dexterity that defies the conventional wisdom surrounding age-related cognitive decline. Through the strategic nourishment of the brain with a symphony of longevity-boosting nutrients, the stimulation of its neuroplastic capacities through intellectual challenges and lifelong learning, and the fortification of its resilience through effective stress management, we have cultivated a level of mental acuity that serves as a beacon of inspiration to all who encounter us.

Gone are the memory lapses, diminished focus, and neurological vulnerabilities that can sometimes accompany growing older. In their place, we exude an intellectual prowess – a problem-solving ability, a creative flair, and an insatiable curiosity that propel us to continually push the boundaries of what is possible.

Robust Emotional Resilience

The embrace of the ageless mindset has also empowered us to cultivate a level of emotional resilience and psychological well-being that defies the challenges often associated with the aging process. Through the integration of effective stress management practices, the nourishment of supportive social connections, and the tapping into a profound sense of purpose and meaning, we have fortified our ability to navigate life's inevitable ups and downs with grace, clarity, and an unwavering sense of inner strength.

Gone are the mood disturbances, anxiety, and depression that can sometimes characterize the later stages of life. In their place, we exude a palpable aura of inner peace, joy, and a profound appreciation for the richness of life – an emotional maturity and adaptability that inspires all who come into our orbit.

A Profound Zest for Living

Perhaps most profoundly, the embrace of the ageless mindset has empowered us to reclaim a profound zest for living – a childlike sense of wonder, curiosity, and a boundless enthusiasm for the endless possibilities that await us, even as the years accumulate. By shedding the limiting beliefs and societal narratives that can often shroud the aging process in fear and trepidation, we have cultivated a bold, visionary perspective that celebrates growing older as a dynamic journey of transformation, reinvention, and the continual expansion of our capabilities and vitality.

Gone is the resignation, complacency, or resignation that can sometimes characterize the later stages of life. In their place, we exude a vibrant, purpose-driven energy – an excitement, anticipation, and a deep, abiding zest for the richness that life has to offer, at every stage of our journey.

The Ripple Effect of Boundless Vitality

As we embrace the life of boundless vitality that has blossomed within us, it becomes clear that the transformative impact of our journey extends far beyond the confines of our own personal experience. Rather, it radiates outwards, creating a powerful ripple effect that has the potential to inspire and uplift all who come into our orbit.

Becoming Beacons of Inspiration

Through the embodiment of our boundless vitality – the radiant energy, the sharp cognitive abilities, the emotional resilience, and the profound zest for living – we become living, breathing examples of what is truly possible when we dare to defy the limitations of age and reclaim our birthright to a life of vibrant, youthful health.

In the eyes of those around us, our very presence becomes a beacon of inspiration – a tangible manifestation of the boundless potential that resides within each and every one of us, regardless of our chronological age. We challenge the conventional wisdom, shatter the societal narratives, and ignite the imaginations of all who witness the remarkable transformation we have undergone.

Cultivating a Multigenerational Legacy of Vitality

As the ripple effect of our boundless vitality continues to expand, it becomes clear that the impact of our journey extends far beyond the confines of our own individual experience. Rather, it has the power to catalyze a multigenerational legacy of vitality, inspiring and empowering successive generations to embrace the ageless mindset and unlock the secrets to a life of boundless energy, sharp cognitive abilities, and a profound zest for living.

Through the sharing of our personal stories, the imparting of our hard-won wisdom, and the embodied example of our remarkable transformation, we become catalysts for a profound cultural shift – one that challenges the limiting beliefs and societal narratives that have so often defined the aging process and redefines the very essence of what it means to grow old.

The Time Is Now: A Call to Boundless Vitality

As we reach the culmination of our comprehensive exploration of the age-defying nutrition plan and the transformative power of the ageless mindset, it is with a profound sense of gratitude, awe, and unwavering determination that we embrace the boundless vitality that now courses through our being.

The time has come to step boldly into this new chapter, to shed the limitations of the past, and to reclaim our birthright to a life of vibrant, youthful health that defies the very passage of time. For in the embrace of our boundless vitality, we become the architects of a bold, visionary future – one where the human spirit soars to new heights, where the boundaries of what is possible are continually pushed, and where the very essence of growing old is redefined, celebrated, and revered.

Let us be the trailblazers, the visionaries, and the living, breathing embodi-ments of this remarkable transformation. Let us inspire and uplift all who cross our paths, igniting the imaginations of generations to come and ushering in a new era of vibrant, youthful health that becomes the new norm, rather than the exception.

The journey has been long, the challenges have been many, but the rewards are beyond measure. For in the embrace of our boundless vitality, we have unlocked the keys to a life of purpose, passion, and a profound zest for living that will echo through the ages, inspiring and empowering all who have the privilege of bearing witness to the remarkable transformation we have undergone.

The time is now. The boundless vitality awaits, beckoning us to step boldly into this new chapter, to unleash the full magnificence of our human potential, and to forge a future where the very essence of aging is redefined, celebrated, and revered.

Let us rise to the challenge, for the vision we hold in our hearts is ours to manifest, one empowered choice at a time. Let us be the beacons of inspiration, the architects of a new narrative, and the living, breathing embodiments of what is truly possible when we dare to defy the limitations of time and reclaim our birthright to a life of boundless vitality.